# TRANSDIAGNOSTIC GROUP THERAPY TRAINING AND IMPLEMENTATION

ELSEVIER

ELSEVIER *science & technology books*

*Companion Web Site:*

**http://store.elsevier.com/product.jsp?&isbn=9780128139899**

***Transdiagnostic Group Therapy Training and Implementation: The Take Control Course***

*Lydia Morris; Warren Mansell; Phil McEvoy; Rachel Bates; Tanya Wallwork; Jody Comiskey*

Resources:

- Videos and slides

ELSEVIER

ACADEMIC PRESS

# TRANSDIAGNOSTIC GROUP THERAPY TRAINING AND IMPLEMENTATION

## The Take Control Course


*Written by*

LYDIA MORRIS
*University of Manchester, Manchester, United Kingdom*

PHIL MCEVOY
*Six Degrees Social Enterprise, Salford, United Kingdom*

TANYA WALLWORK
*Six Degrees Social Enterprise, Salford, United Kingdom*

RACHEL BATES
*Six Degrees Social Enterprise, Salford, United Kingdom*

JODY COMISKEY
*Six Degrees Social Enterprise, Salford, United Kingdom*

WARREN MANSELL
*University of Manchester, Manchester, United Kingdom*



ELSEVIER

ACADEMIC PRESS
An imprint of Elsevier

Academic Press is an imprint of Elsevier
125 London Wall, London EC2Y 5AS, United Kingdom
525 B Street, Suite 1800, San Diego, CA 92101-4495, United States
50 Hampshire Street, 5th Floor, Cambridge, MA 02139, United States
The Boulevard, Langford Lane, Kidlington, Oxford OX5 1GB, United Kingdom



**British Library Cataloguing-in-Publication Data**
A catalogue record for this book is available from the British Library

**Library of Congress Cataloging-in-Publication Data**
A catalog record for this book is available from the Library of Congress

ISBN: 978-0-12-813989-9

For Information on all Academic Press publications
visit our website at https://www.elsevier.com/books-and-journals



*Publisher:* Nikki Levy
*Acquisition Editor:* Nikki Levy
*Editorial Project Manager:* Barbara Makinster
*Production Project Manager:* Anusha Sambamoorthy
*Cover Designer:* Matthew Limbert

Typeset by MPS Limited, Chennai, India

# Contents


**List of Tables** xi
**Biographies** xiii
**Preface** xv
**Acknowledgments** xxi

## PART A

### 1. Introduction to This Book and the Take Control Course 3

Introduction to This Book 3
Why We Have Developed the Take Control Course? 3
Key Points 7
References 7
Further Reading 10

### 2. Conceptual and Theoretical Background 11

Common Processes Across Disorders 11
Introduction to Perceptual Control Theory 12
Summary 19
Key points 21
References 21

### 3. PCT Within Psychological Interventions 23

Perceptual Control Theory Applied Within Individual Interventions 23
Research Focusing on the Take Control Course 25
Components of the Take Control Course (Including the Rationale Based on PCT) 26
Key Points 28
References 29
Further Reading 30

4. How to Use This Book 31

Who is the Take Control Course for? 31
Using This Book 32
How to Organize a Course 37
Key Points 40
References 40

# PART B

5. Session 1 Thinking About Control 45

Overview 45
Key Session Focus 45
Overall Rationale 46
Before the Session 51
Session Sections (Overview and Steps 1–3) 52
How to Take Control (Step 4 Onwards) 64
Steps 6 and 7: Goal-Focused Exposure Technique 68
All Materials Required 74
Do not Forget! 74
End of Chapter Quiz 75
Condensed Session Plan: Session 1 75
Awareness Exercise Prompts 76
Guided Exposure in Imagination Prompts 77
References 77

6. Session 2 What Blocks Our Control? 79

Overview 79
Key Session Focus 79
Overall Rationale 80
Rationale: PCA Problem-Solving Tool 82
Before the Session 83
Session Sections 84
Materials Required 93
Don't Forget 93
End of Chapter Quiz 94
Condensed Session Plan: Session 2 94
Awareness Exercise Prompts 95
Guided Exposure in Imagination Prompts 95
References 96

7. Session 3 Feeling in Control Short Term vs Getting Control of Your Life 97

Overview 97
Key Session Focus 97
Overall Rationale: Hierarchies Revisited 98
Rationale: Understanding Emotions 99
Before the Session 101
Session Sections 101
Materials Required 107
Don't Forget 108
End of Chapter Quiz 108
Condensed Session Plan: Session 3 109
Body Awareness 109
Guided Exposure in Imagination Prompts 110
References 111

8. Session 4 Taking Control of the Things Around You 113

Overview 113
Key Session Focus 113
Overall Rationale 114
Rationale: Is Conflict Always Unhelpful? 117
Before the Session 118
Session Sections 118
Materials Required 132
Don't Forget 133
End of Chapter Quiz 133
Condensed Session Plan: Session 4 134
Session 4: Guided Exposure in Imagination Prompts 135
Guided Exposure in Imagination Prompts 135
References 136

9. Session 5 Building on Strengths, Qualities, and Resources 137

Overview 137
Key Session Focus 137
Overall Rationale 138
Before the Session 140
Session Sections 141
Materials Required 146
End of Chapter Quiz 146
Condensed Session Plan: Session 5 147
Compassionate Awareness 147
References 149

10. Session 6 Moving Forward: What Gets Me Stuck, What Helps 151

Overview 151
Key Session Focus 151
Overall Rationale 152
Rationale: Using the "Imagination Mode" 153
Before the Session 153
Session Sections 154
Materials Required 159
Condensed Session Plan: Session 6 160
References 160

PART C

11. Riding the Waves of Cognitive Behavioral Therapy: Contextualizing the Take Control Course Within Cognitive Behavioral Therapy 163

The History of the Development of Transdiagnostic Cognitive Behavioral Therapy 164
The Conceptual Basis of Third Wave Transdiagnostic Approaches 165
Evidence for Third Wave and Transdiagnostic Interventions 167
Interim Summary 171
Distinctiveness and Overlap With Other Transdiagnostic Approaches 171
Summary and Conclusions 176
References 177

12. Embracing the Diversity Within the Course: Revisiting Theory and Practice to Address Clients' Personal Concerns 183

Chronic Lack of Control 185
Limited Awareness of Higher Level Goals 190
The Uniqueness of Each Client's Problems 194
Summary 198
References 200

13. Taking Practice Forward 201

Developing Your Practice 201
Evaluating Your Practice 202
Adapting the Take Control Course 202
References 204
Useful Websites 204
Further Reading 204

Appendix A: Accessibility, Clarity, and Ease of Use of the Take Control Course Manual: A Qualitative Study 205
Appendix B: Overview of All the Sessions 211
Appendix C: Sessional Evaluation Form 215
Appendix D: Take Control Course: Competence and Adherence Scale 219
Appendix E: Session Guides for All Sessions (1–6) 225
Appendix F: Possible Metaphors to Use With Awareness Exercise 239
Index 241

For additional information on the topics covered in the book, visit the companion site: http://store.elsevier.com/product.jsp?&isbn=9780128139899

# List of Tables


| | | |
|---|---|---|
| Table 2.1 | Summary of Key Perceptual Control Theory (PCT) Terms Used | 12 |
| Table 11.1 | Key Principles of PCT and Examples of Similarities/ Differences to Familiar Psychotherapies | 174 |
| Table 12.1 | The Themes of This Chapter Are Recapped in the Summary Table | 199 |

# Biographies

The author team includes established academics and clinicians. Clinicians from varied backgrounds are represented, including Clinical Psychology and Mental Health Nursing. Dr. Morris, Dr. McEvoy, and Dr. Mansell have considerable clinical experience in primary care contexts and have authored papers and books contributing to the field of transdiagnostic research.

Dr. Lydia Morris is a Clinical Psychologist who has extensive experience of working in mental health primary care contexts. The manual was in part written while Dr. Morris was employed by Manchester Mental Health and Social Care Trust. She has been affiliated with the University of Manchester for much of the duration of the manual production and is now employed by the University of Salford.

Dr. Phil McEvoy is service director of a primary care team (Six Degrees Social Enterprise, Salford, Greater Manchester). Six Degrees Social Enterprise delivers socially innovative mental health services that are at the leading edge of practice. In recent years they have been finalists in the National Positive Practice in Mental Health Awards, the National Patient Experience Awards, and the Health Service Journal Awards.

Dr. Warren Mansell is a highly regarded researcher, who has authored a number of texts on psychological approaches. These include: *Cognitive Behavioral Processes Across Disorders* (Harvey, Watkins, Mansell & Shafran, 2004); a self-help book called *Coping with fears and phobias: a step-by-step guide to understanding and facing your anxieties* (Mansell, 2007); and a number of therapy manuals (Mansell, Carey & Tai, 2013; Carey, Mansell & Tai, 2015; Stott et al., 2010), including *Transdiagnostic CBT using Method of Levels Therapy* (Mansell, Carey, & Tai, 2013). He has been employed by the University of Manchester throughout the duration of the manual production.

Ms. Wallwork, Tanya; Comiskey, Jody; and Bates, Rachel are all clinicians who were working within the Six Degrees primary care team during the development of the Take Control Course and production of this manual. They all worked in this context for over 6 years. They have provided input regarding the relevance of the material to the clients they work with and the context they work within. They have also contributed to the development of supplementary resources, e.g., training videos.

# Preface

We, the authors, see this manual as a wonderful opportunity. We have been working together on designing, delivering, training facilitators, and evaluating the Take Control Course for many years now. Our own professions span clinical psychology, clinical research, mental health nursing, and management. Our clinical experience ranges from so-called "low intensity" psychological interventions to so-called "severe mental illness."

Despite this wide range of backgrounds and clients, we have each been consistently struck by some basic facts about how people get "stuck," and how they get themselves out of being "stuck." Each individual we meet is *unique*, with their own personal story, their own values and private difficulties, and their own array of ways that they cope and eventually recover. On the face of it, problems such as an eating disorder, chronic panic attacks, anger issues, and depression might look very different. Yet, at the same time, we have seen that the problems of every person seem to boil down to the same basic pattern. Patients come to us because they have lost control of an important aspect of their lives. Through curious questioning we typically find that this stems from an unresolved dilemma that has remained unchanged because the client has never freely expressed the root of their difficulties. As we provide an opportunity for the client to express their problems in this way and contemplate their issues at length and in depth, a remarkable process happens. The client starts to have their own insights and make their own choices, and eventually, these have a real, tangible difference in their lives.

You may be aware that there is a psychological therapy known as method of levels (MOL) that aims to distill this universal experience and help people resolve their distress. We each practice MOL and use it with our own clients for individual therapy. But we soon recognized that we were missing an opportunity. How could we help more people access it? Could we manage it by demonstrating the underlying principles of MOL, and setting up the conditions for people to use them in their own lives? We do use MOL when we talk to clients during the Take Control Course. But clearly this is unrealistic in a large group and it is hard (but not impossible) to do individual therapy without personal disclosure. While we recognized that some people will be happy with personal disclosure in a group, others would not. What is more, if the most important element of change is freely exploring one's own problems, regardless of who listens, can we help people make the changes they need without individual therapy?

The aim of the Take Control Course has therefore always been to try to bottle the ingredients of this recovery process, and share it widely. Our hope is that a brief group course can provide the chance to think about one's own life in terms of simple, shared principles. For some people, this might be all they need to reach a turning point in their lives and make the change they need. For many the course complements the help they have received so far, and will later receive. Our research with clients who have done the course seems to support our hopes, and so, it seems appropriate, or even essential, that we help other services run the course too. We have seen the course being taken up for a wide range of patient groups—across ages and beyond mental health services—which has encouraged us further.

One thing you might need to come to terms with as you read the manual is that it is a *theory-based* manual. To be specific, *every* element of the course, including why and how you talk to the clients during the course, is theory driven. That is not to say you cannot be yourself and have a chat when people are looking for a place to hang their coat when they arrive! It also does not mean you have to be a perfect Take Control Course facilitator when you start—you will need to draw on your own intuition and your wider training at times. What it does mean is that there is one, simple model for why we think the course should be helpful people. That model is perceptual control theory.

All the science will be explained clearly later. Here we want to reassure you that this theory can be easily and readily understood. In fact, at the level you need to understand it for the course, it is not complicated at all. But it is different from what you are used to. And it does challenge some of the assumptions that other psychological treatments have. We think this is exactly how it should be. If we are to try to extract the common features of recovery from a mental health problem, regardless of the diagnosis and regardless of the particular technique or demographic of the client, then that theory will need to be novel.

We would like to sum up three major differences you might expect here, so you are prepared for what comes later, and you can see how much this manual will genuinely appeal to you. So here goes!

1. *Everything a person does is part of their attempt to try to control some kind of experience they are having*—to see, hear, feel, and perceive themselves and people around them in a certain way. In fact, we are so focused on getting the experience we want, that we may be completely unaware of *how* we are doing it, and what this looks like to other people. So, in the Take Control Course, we do not expect

people to be aware of what *we* can see them doing—but to be aware of what personal experience they are striving for. If a client mentions their "avoidance" or their "obsessive behaviour" or their "panic," we want to help them focus on what they wanted to experience at the time—what was the underlying "goal" or "ideal." It might be to feel safe, to feel dominant, or to suppress a distressing memory—only the client can know. As a facilitator, we do not have our own agenda for whether that behavior itself should change, or whether it is a good or bad thing. The behavior is just part of a bigger, more important whole—to control something.

2. *Only the individual client can determine whether something they are doing is a problem for them.* Any action whether private or public is only a problem to the extent that it takes someone away from an experience that the person wants (or someone who they value wants). All problems are relative problems. Tim Carey has likened this to a psychological "law or relativity." There are no "dysfunctional" behaviors or thoughts or attitudes. Worry is sometimes useful to help think of possible future problems to be averted. Suppressing one's own emotions helps a person manage in many challenging jobs. Making a fool of yourself is the whole point if you are a clown or a comedian. The problem comes with the *conflict*. Worry makes me more anxious than I can cope with; pushing away my emotions at home makes me feel estranged from my family; making a fool of myself at work makes others doubt my competence. Taking this on board a facilitator on the course treats every term—that people might assume is an issue—at face value. When the topic of worry, for example, is brought up and a client states "I need to stop worrying," we ask, "How bothered are you about worrying?," or "How much worry is OK?" or "When you stop worrying would you ever want to start it again?" We do not assume that stop worrying is the aim of the course for this or any other clients.
3. *Change happens in its own time.* When running the course, not only do we not try to change people's behavior. We also do not try to change their goals. In fact, we do not even encourage people to change their own goals. This might seem quite passive. What are we doing then? To put it simply, we are giving people a chance to broaden their awareness; to *discover* their own needs, goals, and values, and importantly, how they are all related to one another in their everyday lives. On the Take Control Course, we manage this in large groups by explaining the basic concepts of perceptual control theory in easy, accessible, and sometimes fun, ways. In individual therapy, this is often not necessary of course because the therapist can gear their questions around the client. Yet the aim of MOL, the individual therapy we draw on in the course, is the same as within the Take

Control Course—to broaden awareness. We focus purely on this partly because it is guided by theory, but also because we have seen that this is one of the most important experiences that clients say they get from *any* psychological intervention. And ethically, we want our clients to be in control of their own choices. The funny thing is that, ultimately, change itself is not fully governed by the person. It comes and goes, ideas pop into people's heads, and people "find themselves" doing something that makes a positive difference. This is not how the Take Control Course causes change. This is how change happens regardless of what helped it happen. In the theory it is called *reorganization* and we revisit this idea regularly.

So, if you are OK with the idea that you will not be advising people to behave or think differently after this course, if you embrace the idea that change is something we cannot control the timing of, and you can put your own judgements to one side to be curious at all times, then the Take Control Course is the course for you. Or may be you think you are interested in whether going down these lines *might* be helpful because you simply *need* to deliver an intervention to a wider group of patients in large numbers, and you can see that a diagnosis is not required, then please read on. We hope to present you with more than enough information to decide this for yourself by the end of the book, or once you have tried it out.

This book is written in three parts. The first part sets the stage for the course by explaining why we think it is needed in services, what is the background theory and its use in mental health interventions to date, and how to use this book. In the second part, we describe each session of the course in detail. We provide objectives for each session, slides, worksheets, vignettes, session plans, key points, and self-test questions for each session. We have collected feedback from clinicians over the course of writing this manual and have incorporated their feedback and suggestions, such as offering a self-test or quiz (for more details of this evaluation project see Appendix A: Accessibility, Clarity and Ease of Use of the Take Control Course Manual: A Qualitative Study). In the third part, we provide more details on MOL therapy, and we share with you ideas of how you might take the practice of the Take Control Course and PCT forward, including what you might consider if you want to adapt it for a wider audience.

As we said at the start, we (the authors) have diverse backgrounds, and we would like to help diverse professionals and helpers of all backgrounds to use this course. It is not a course that can be delivered without a good understanding of its principles, some particular skills in how to ask questions, and a good knowledge of the materials. We have included ways throughout the manual for you to try to judge this for yourself. But if you feel you need to contact one of us about any aspect of this course and who it might be helpful for, then please do. We want to encourage a healthy and critical discussion. Feedback from clients and clinicians has been essential in the development of the Take Control Course to date, and we see this as the case going forward to. We hope that you now have a manual that is "fit for purpose" and that putting it into practice is rewarding and valuable, and even fun and enlightening at times! Now, you take control...

# Acknowledgments

We would firstly like to thank the innovator of the Perceptual Control Theory—William T. Powers—for his groundbreaking and tireless work. We are very grateful for all the effort developing this theory that so informs our work. We are also very grateful to the team at Six Degrees Social Enterprise—some of whom have been involved in developing this manuscript. So many individuals within this team have directly and indirectly supported research into the Take Control Course. As well as those who have been involved in authoring this manual, we want to thank Rachel Ukeles, Debra Frazer, and Greg Dove for their support in producing the videos for this manual and in developing the course.

Many thanks to Prof. Kent McClelland, Prof. Tim Carey, Dr. Elizabeth Murphy, Dr. Sally Higginson, and again the team members at Six Degrees Social Enterprise for their feedback regarding the content of the Take Control Course at the initial stages of development. Many thanks to Derek Marriott for the presentation and content advice on the Take Control Course materials. We would also like to acknowledge and thank Zoe Hayden for her fantastic cartoons.

We would like to thank the academics that have particularly supported the research into Take Control Course: Prof. Richard Emsley, Prof. Karina Lovell, and Dr. Dawn Edge. Dr. Sara Tai and Dr. Vyv Huddy have also provided useful feedback regarding the research program. We are also grateful to the people who participated in the studies, and all those who enabled the research. Many thanks to Rebekah Warke, Martina Slapkova, Saoirse Kennedy-Barton, Amel Hamlaoui, and Rebekah Amos (research assistants on some of the research studies).

# PART A

CHAPTER

# 1

# Introduction to This Book and the Take Control Course

## INTRODUCTION TO THIS BOOK

This book describes a group-based intervention called the Take Control Course. Chapters 2-4 provide background to the development Course and information about how to set up a Course. Subsequent chapters provide a detailed overview of each of the six sessions of the Course. The final section of the book (Part C) focuses on ways that facilitators can enhance their delivery of the Take Control Course.

## WHY WE HAVE DEVELOPED THE TAKE CONTROL COURSE?

There are many Cognitive Behavioral interventions already available with a substantial number of research studies showing that these are effective (Butler, Chapman, Forman, & Beck, 2006; Hofmann, Asnaani, Vonk, Sawyer, & Fang, 2012; Hunsley & Lee, 2007; Stewart & Chambless, 2009). However, a number of large surveys indicate that many people do not receive psychological treatment even for common mental health problems, such as anxiety and depression (Alonso et al., 2004; Wang et al., 2005, 2007; Young, Klap, Sherbourne, & Wells, 2001). This suggests that there needs to be greater access to evidence-based psychological interventions. Psychological interventions need to be cost-effective in order to make it more likely that they can be made readily available. One of the reasons for the way we have developed the Take Control Course is on the basis of pragmatic reasons, such as cost-effectiveness, but there are a number of other equally important

*Transdiagnostic Group Therapy Training and Implementation*
DOI: https://doi.org/10.1016/B978-0-12-813989-9.00001-4

theoretical reasons why the Take Control Course has been developed in the way that it has. These reasons are summarized in this chapter.

## Because Some Clients Can Get "Added Value" From Groups

A number of studies indicate that some clients can derive particular benefits from engaging in group interventions. For example, these include normalization of experience, "other people are having the same struggles as me," and interpersonal support, "the group context helped me to keep trying out techniques and persevering" (e.g., Finucane & Mercer, 2006; Mason & Hargreaves, 2001). Clearly this does not mean that groups are the best option for everyone, but groups can offer a useful alternative to individual interventions.

## To Target Common Processes Across Disorders

Until fairly recently many of the Cognitive Behavioral interventions available have been offered, as a manualized protocol, to clients with one specific disorder. For example, specific protocols have been developed to be offered to clients with Social Anxiety Disorder, which is characterized by a fear of social situations and being around people (Clark et al., 2003; Stangier, Heidenreich, Peitz, Lauterbach, & Clark, 2003; Wells, 1997). These target cognitive and behavioral processes that have been found to contribute to psychological distress and problematic symptoms in this disorder. For example, some interventions for social anxiety target the way in which clients can focus on themselves in social situations and can miss positive external cues, because this has been shown to contribute to problematic symptoms (Hirsch & Mathews, 2000; Hofmann, 2007).

However, more and more research has shown that many of these processes contribute to psychological distress across a number of disorders; for example, worry and other repetitive thinking occur in a number of anxiety and depressive disorders (Harvey, Watkins, Mansell, & Shafran, 2004; Nolen-Hoeksema & Watkins, 2011). Processes that occur across a number of disorders are described as transdiagnostic. In addition to this support for the transdiagnostic nature of such processes, often when people seek help for distressing symptoms it is possible to describe their symptoms using more than one disorder label (described as comorbidity) (e.g., Jenkins et al., 2009). Conversely, sometimes it is hard to give people a specific disorder label, as their symptoms do not fit neatly under a particular label. Therefore researchers have started to design and research transdiagnostic interventions because such interventions can target the processes that contribute to symptoms that could be categorized under different disorder labels. Such interventions offer the potential to develop generalizable clinician skills; for example, using conceptualizations and techniques that are readily adapted for clients with comorbid or unusual problems (Alexander, Arnkoff, & Glass, 2010; McHugh & Barlow, 2010; Richards & Bower, 2011; Shafran et al., 2009).

There are a number of journal articles and other resources that describe the evidence base and rationale for a transdiagnostic approach (e.g., Harvey et al., 2004; Mansell, Harvey, Watkins, & Shafran, 2009; Nolen-Hoeksema & Watkins, 2011). For those who are interested, there are also a number of articles that provide neurobiological research that supports a transdiagnostic approach (e.g., Buckholtz & Meyer-Lindenberg, 2012; Goschke, 2014).

## To Offer More Cost-Effective Interventions

Overall the majority of research studies that compared individual and group interventions have found that groups are more cost-effective than individual therapy; however, there are limits to the available studies (Tucker & Oei, 2007). Although a substantial number of studies have compared the cost-effectiveness of groups and individual psychological interventions, only a minority of studies have included broader societal costs (Tucker & Oei, 2007). For example, the majority of studies have focused on costs to health care providers and few have factored in the costs to clients that could be incurred from missing work to attend fixed-time group sessions (Tucker & Oei, 2007; Wolff, Helminiak, & Tebes, 1997). We have focused particularly heavily on the research basis in regards to this because it seems to make intuitive sense that groups would be more cost-effective (as you can see more people at once). In particular the Take Control Course is designed to be delivered to large groups, as it does not rely on interactions between members of the group.

## To Allow Clients to Attend Sessions in a Flexible Way

An explicit emphasis of the Take Control Course is that clients can choose which sessions they attend; for example, they might chose not to attend a session that does not seem so relevant to their problems. There is increasing evidence that psychological change occurs at a different pace and in a varied ways for different people. For example, there is evidence that some clients can experience "sudden gains" (can be described as eureka/aha moments, insights, etc.) that contribute a significant amount to their improvement by the end of the intervention (Aderka, Nickerson, Bøe, & Hofmann, 2012; Norton, Klenck, & Barrera, 2010; Tang & DeRubeis, 1999). Hayes, Laurenceau, Feldman, Strauss, and Cardaciotto (2007) reviewed a number of different strands of research that illustrate psychological change that is not linear and gradual. For example, studies suggest that anxiety and distress levels can increase before symptoms improve. Another example is from the research looking at responses to traumatic events. Some people experience posttraumatic stress disorder (PTSD), others could experience personal growth (in terms of changes in life priorities and greater personal strength, etc.), while others could experience both PTSD and personal growth (Tedeschi & Calhoun, 2004).

Clinicians and researchers commonly offer clients a set number of sessions, e.g., 6 or 8 or 15. Such clinical practice is often informed by research studies but generally the number of sessions offered in research studies is not based on what is most effective. For example, demonstrating that 12 weekly sessions are an effective time frame does not demonstrate that this is the most effective time frame or that 12 sessions is actually required. It is understandable that treatments are often specified in this way but in routine clinical practice clients often do not attend the specified number of sessions (Barkham et al., 2006; Glover, Webb, & Evison, 2010). It is possible that clients are "voting with their feet" and letting us know that the prescribed number of sessions is not always what they find most useful. This makes sense given the research indicating that change happens at a different pace for different people. It has been suggested that, in clinical practice, clients and clinicians regulate their treatment attendance on an ongoing basis and continue treatment until they have achieved a personally "good enough" level of change (Barkham et al., 2006; Stiles, Barkham, Connell, & Mellor-Clark, 2008).

One of the concerns about allowing clients to choose the number of sessions that they attend is that people will attend an unmanageable number. However, a number of studies (across different clinical settings) that have allowed clients to choose the sessions they attend have found that clients generally attend a low average number of sessions, such as between four and six (Mansell, Carey, & Tai, 2012), although a few clients may access a larger number the majority attends a small number (Carey, 2005; Carey, Tai, & Stiles, 2013). Dramatic improvements in waiting times, access to services and missed/canceled appointments have been observed using this "client-led" approach (e.g., Carey & Spratt, 2009). The Take Control Course has been specifically designed to allow that clients may not need to, or be able to, attend every session. It can also be offered using a *rolling format*, which is discussed in more detail in Part C, Chapter 3.

## Accessible Format and Style

The theoretical framework that underpins the course allows us to focus on a small number of simple concepts that we have found ring true with clients. Naturally the key tenet is "control." Clients are very familiar with their struggles to control aspects of their lives and they tend to find the tasks around understanding control very engaging. In contrast, some clients struggle to label their thoughts and feelings, especially at the start of a psychological intervention. The Take Control Course does not necessarily require participants to label their thoughts, feelings, behavior, attitudes, and assumptions, as might be necessary for a classic CBT course. The interpersonal style of the facilitators also promotes accessibility because they are attuned to the importance of helping group members maintain adequate control and feel safe in the group setting.

## KEY POINTS

- Some people seem to get added value from groups.
- Groups have generally been found to be more cost-effective than individual interventions.
- Increasing research suggests that disorder categorizations may not be the most helpful way to understand psychological distress.
- Transdiagnostic interventions are ones that target processes that maintain psychological distress across disorders.
- Enabling clients to choose how many sessions they attend can be beneficial for the clients and the service.

## References

Aderka, I. M., Nickerson, A., Bøe, H. J., & Hofmann, S. G. (2012). Sudden gains during psychological treatments of anxiety and depression: A meta-analysis. *Journal of consulting and clinical psychology, 80*(1), 93. Available from https://doi.org/10.1037/a0026455.

Alexander, C. L., Arnkoff, D. B., & Glass, C. R. (2010). Bringing psychotherapy to primary care: Innovations and challenges. *Clinical Psychology: Science and Practice, 17*(3), 191–214. Available from https://doi.org/10.1111/j.1468-2850.2010.01211.x.

Alonso, J., Angermeyer, M. C., Bernert, S., Bruffaerts, R., Brugha, T., Bryson, H., ... Gasquet, I. (2004). Use of mental health services in Europe: Results from the European Study of the Epidemiology of Mental Disorders (ESEMeD) project. *Acta Psychiatrica Scandinavica, 109*(s420), 47–54. Available from https://doi.org/10.1111/j.1600-0047.2004.00329.x.

Barkham, M., Connell, J., Stiles, W. B., Miles, J. N., Margison, F., Evans, C., & Mellor-Clark, J. (2006). Dose-effect relations and responsive regulation of treatment duration: The good enough level. *Journal of Consulting and Clinical Psychology, 74*(1), 160. Available from https://doi.org/10.1037/0022-006X.74.1.160.

Buckholtz, J. W., & Meyer-Lindenberg, A. (2012). Psychopathology and the human connectome: Toward a transdiagnostic model of risk for mental illness. *Neuron, 74*(6), 990–1004. Available from https://doi.org/10.1016/j.neuron.2012.06.002.

Butler, A. C., Chapman, J. E., Forman, E. M., & Beck, A. T. (2006). The empirical status of cognitive-behavioral therapy: A review of meta-analyses. *Clinical Psychology Review, 26*(1), 17–31. Available from https://doi.org/10.1016/j.cpr.2005.07.003.

Carey, T. A. (2005). Can patients specify treatment parameters? A preliminary investigation. *Clinical Psychology & Psychotherapy, 12*(4), 326–335. Available from https://doi.org/10.1002/cpp.455.

Carey, T. A., & Spratt, M. B. (2009). When is enough enough? Structuring the organisation of treatment to maximise patient choice and control. *The Cognitive Behaviour Therapist, 2*, 211–226. Available from https://doi.org/10.1017/S1754470X09000208.

Carey, T. A., Tai, S. J., & Stiles, W. B. (2013). Effective and efficient: Using patient-led appointment scheduling in routine mental health practice in remote Australia. *Professional Psychology: Research and Practice, 44*(6), 405. Available from https://doi.org/10.1037/a0035038.

Clark, D. M., Ehlers, A., McManus, F., Hackmann, A., Fennell, M., Campbell, H., ... Louis, B. (2003). Cognitive therapy versus fluoxetine in generalized social phobia: A randomized placebo-controlled trial. *Journal of Consulting and Clinical Psychology, 71*(6), 1058.

Finucane, A., & Mercer, S. W. (2006). An exploratory mixed methods study of the acceptability and effectiveness of mindfulness-based cognitive therapy for patients with active depression and anxiety in primary care. *BMC Psychiatry, 6*(1), 14. Available from https://doi.org/10.1186/1471-244X-6-14.

Glover, G., Webb, M., & Evison, F. (2010). Improving access to psychological therapies: A review of the progress made by sites in the first roll-out year. *North East Public Health Observatory.* <http://www.iapt.nhs.uk/silo/files/iapt-a-review-of-the-progress-made-by-sites-in-the-first-roll8208-out-year.pdf>.

Goschke, T. (2014). Dysfunctions of decision-making and cognitive control as transdiagnostic mechanisms of mental disorders: Advances, gaps, and needs in current research. *International Journal of Methods in Psychiatric Research, 23*(S1), 41–57. Available from https://doi.org/10.1002/mpr.1410.

Harvey, A. G., Watkins, E., Mansell, W., & Shafran, R. (2004). *Cognitive behavioural processes across psychological disorders: A transdiagnostic approach to research and treatment.* USA: Oxford University Press.

Hayes, A. M., Laurenceau, J.-P., Feldman, G., Strauss, J. L., & Cardaciotto, L. (2007). Change is not always linear: The study of nonlinear and discontinuous patterns of change in psychotherapy. *Clinical Psychology Review, 27*(6), 715–723. Available from https://doi.org/10.1016/j.cpr.2007.01.008.

Hirsch, C. R., & Mathews, A. (2000). Impaired positive inferential bias in social phobia. *Journal of Abnormal Psychology, 109*(4), 705.

Hofmann, S. G. (2007). Cognitive factors that maintain social anxiety disorder: A comprehensive model and its treatment implications. *Cognitive Behaviour Therapy, 36*(4), 193–209. Available from https://doi.org/10.1080/16506070701421313.

Hofmann, S. G., Asnaani, A., Vonk, I. J., Sawyer, A. T., & Fang, A. (2012). The efficacy of cognitive behavioral therapy: A review of meta-analyses. *Cognitive Therapy and Research, 36*(5), 427–440. Available from https://doi.org/10.1007/s10608-012-9476-1.

Hunsley, J., & Lee, C. M. (2007). Research-informed benchmarks for psychological treatments: Efficacy studies, effectiveness studies, and beyond. *Professional Psychology: Research and Practice, 38*(1), 21. Available from https://doi.org/10.1037/0735-7028.38.1.21.

Jenkins, R., Meltzer, H., Bebbington, P., Brugha, T., Farrell, M., McManus, S., & Singleton, N. (2009). The British mental health survey programme: Achievements and latest findings. *Social Psychiatry and Psychiatric Epidemiology, 44*(11), 899–904. Available from https://doi.org/10.1007/s00127-009-0112-7.

Mansell, W., Carey, T. A., & Tai, S. J. (2012). *A transdiagnostic approach to CBT using method of levels therapy: Distinctive features.* New York: Routledge.

Mansell, W., Harvey, A., Watkins, E., & Shafran, R. (2009). Conceptual foundations of the transdiagnostic approach to CBT. *Journal of Cognitive Psychotherapy, 23*(1), 6–19. Available from https://doi.org/10.1891/0889-8391.23.1.6, [provides an update of transdiagnostic research, considers theoretical accounts that could explain the empirical data].

Mason, O., & Hargreaves, I. (2001). A qualitative study of mindfulness based cognitive therapy for depression. *British Journal of Medical Psychology, 74*, 197–221.

McHugh, R. K., & Barlow, D. H. (2010). The dissemination and implementation of evidence-based psychological treatments: A review of current efforts. *American Psychologist, 65*(2), 73. Available from https://doi.org/10.1037/a0018121.

Nolen-Hoeksema, S., & Watkins, E. R. (2011). A heuristic for developing transdiagnostic models of psychopathology explaining multifinality and divergent trajectories. *Perspectives on Psychological Science, 6*(6), 589–609. Available from https://doi.org/10.1177/1745691611419672.

Norton, P. J., Klenck, S. C., & Barrera, T. L. (2010). Sudden gains during cognitive-behavioral group therapy for anxiety disorders. *Journal of Anxiety Disorders, 24*(8), 887–892. Available from https://doi.org/10.1016/j.janxdis.2010.06.012.

Richards, D. A., & Bower, P. (2011). Equity of access to psychological therapies. *The British Journal of Psychiatry, 198*(2), 91–92. Available from https://doi.org/10.1192/bjp.bp.110.083485.

Shafran, R., Clark, D., Fairburn, C., Arntz, A., Barlow, D., Ehlers, A., ... Ost, L. (2009). Mind the gap: Improving the dissemination of CBT. *Behaviour Research and Therapy, 47* (11), 902–909. Available from https://doi.org/10.1016/j.brat.2009.07.003.

Stangier, U., Heidenreich, T., Peitz, M., Lauterbach, W., & Clark, D. (2003). Cognitive therapy for social phobia: Individual versus group treatment. *Behaviour Research and Therapy, 41*(9), 991–1007.

Stewart, R. E., & Chambless, D. L. (2009). Cognitive–behavioral therapy for adult anxiety disorders in clinical practice: A meta-analysis of effectiveness studies. *Journal of Consulting and Clinical Psychology, 77*(4), 595. Available from https://doi.org/10.1037/a0016032.

Stiles, W. B., Barkham, M., Connell, J., & Mellor-Clark, J. (2008). Responsive regulation of treatment duration in routine practice in United Kingdom primary care settings: Replication in a larger sample. *Journal of Consulting and Clinical Psychology, 76*(2), 298.

Tang, T. Z., & DeRubeis, R. J. (1999). Sudden gains and critical sessions in cognitive-behavioral therapy for depression. *Journal of Consulting and Clinical Psychology, 67*(6), 894. Available from https://doi.org/10.1037/0022-006X.67.6.894.

Tedeschi, R. G., & Calhoun, L. G. (2004). Posttraumatic growth: Conceptual foundations and empirical evidence. *Psychological Inquiry, 15*(1), 1–18. Available from https://doi.org/10.1207/s15327965pli1501_01.

Tucker, M., & Oei, T. P. (2007). Is group more cost effective than individual cognitive behaviour therapy? The evidence is not solid yet. *Behavioural and Cognitive Psychotherapy, 35*(1), 77. Available from https://doi.org/10.1017/S1352465806003134.

Wang, P. S., Aguilar-Gaxiola, S., Alonso, J., Angermeyer, M. C., Borges, G., Bromet, E. J., ... Gureje, O. (2007). Worldwide use of mental health services for anxiety, mood, and substance disorders: Results from 17 countries in the WHO World Mental Health (WMH) Surveys. *Lancet, 370*(9590), 841. Available from https://doi.org/10.1016/S0140-6736(07)61414-7.

Wang, P. S., Lane, M., Olfson, M., Pincus, H. A., Wells, K. B., & Kessler, R. C. (2005). Twelve-month use of mental health services in the United States: Results from the National Comorbidity Survey Replication. *Archives of General Psychiatry, 62*(6), 629. Available from https://doi.org/10.1001/archpsyc.62.6.629.

Wells, A. (1997). *Cognitive therapy of anxiety disorders*. J. Wiley & sons.

Wolff, N., Helminiak, T. W., & Tebes, J. K. (1997). Getting the cost right in cost-effectiveness analyses. *American Journal of Psychiatry, 154*(6), 736–743.

Young, A. S., Klap, R., Sherbourne, C. D., & Wells, K. B. (2001). The quality of care for depressive and anxiety disorders in the United States. *Archives of General Psychiatry, 58* (1), 55–61. Available from https://doi.org/10.1001/archpsyc.58.1.55.

## Further Reading

Harvey, A. G., Watkins, E. R., Mansell, W., & Shafran, R. (2004). *Cognitive behavioural processes across psychological disorders: A transdiagnostic approach to research and treatment.* Oxford, UK: OUP, [provides a systematic review of the research literature which supports a transdiagnostic account].

CHAPTER

# 2

# Conceptual and Theoretical Background

The Take Control Course (TCC) draws from three main strands of research. It draws on research into cognitive behavioral therapy (CBT) and particularly research into the underlying processes that contribute to psychological distress. It is also influenced by research that suggests that some processes contribute to psychological distress and problematic symptoms across a number of different psychological disorders. Finally it draws on Perceptual Control Theory (PCT; Powers, 1973), which is a theory that provides a framework for understanding psychological functioning as a whole and for understanding what contributes for psychological distress.

## COMMON PROCESSES ACROSS DISORDERS

As described in the previous chapter, increasing research has found that certain cognitive and behavioral processes can contribute to psychological distress across psychological disorders. These processes, which are problematic across disorders, are described as transdiagnostic processes.

The TCC is derived from PCT (Powers,1973). PCT is a transdiagnostic theory that proposes generic mechanisms that account for psychological distress across disorders (Higginson, Mansell, & Wood, 2011; Mansell, 2005). These mechanisms are unique to the theory and provide a fundamental ethos for how to provide an intervention. PCT provides an explanation of why certain processes that are proposed by other theories are actually a problem for the individual (described in more detail in the next section). Therefore, the TCC is a transdiagnostic intervention because it targets generic mechanisms according to PCT.

*Transdiagnostic Group Therapy Training and Implementation*
DOI: https://doi.org/10.1016/B978-0-12-813989-9.00002-6

## INTRODUCTION TO PERCEPTUAL CONTROL THEORY

PCT was developed in the 1950s and 1960s and is informed by the field of control engineering (Powers, 1973; Powers, Clark, & Mc Farland, 1960a, 1960b). This section provides a brief overview of PCT and Table 2.1 provides a summary of key terms.

**TABLE 2.1** Summary of Key Perceptual Control Theory (PCT) Terms Used

| Term | Definition | Example |
|---|---|---|
| Reference values or goal | Internal standard that is based on genetic predisposition and/or past experience. *"Goals" and "reference values" refer to a broad range of reference points that encompass values, beliefs, schemas, etc.* | Reference values can be considered as a set of personal "just rights." There is a huge range of possible examples, from reference values for a good cup of coffee (e.g., milky but strong) to reference values for being a good person (e.g., kind, honest, etc.). |
| Control | Keeping a perception as close as possible to a desired reference value | Being a caring friend; keeping feelings of anxiety at zero; living a good life. |
| Error (or discrepancy) | The difference between the wanted and the experienced reference value | Feeling that have let a friend down by not being caring enough; anxiety more than can tolerate; feeling not living life as wanted. |
| Control hierarchy (system) | Internal reference values that are arranged in a hierarchical network | Each individual will have a multitude of hierarchies. Higher-level goals (e.g., the self-concept of being successful) leading to the setting of subgoals for an individual's principles (e.g., achieving at work), which in turn regulate lower-level, shorter-term goals (e.g., working long hours). |
| (Goal) conflict | The state when two control systems attempt to control an experience with respect to two (or more) opposing reference values | Carey (2008) gives this example of a client who presented with depression, indecisiveness, and lack of sense of purpose. The client had a conflict between reference values of a child self that is spontaneous and reckless and a parent self that has duties. Both the "child self" and "parent self" values would often apply to the same decision or behavior. |

*(Continued)*

TABLE 2.1 (Continued)

| Term | Definition | Example |
|---|---|---|
| Reorganization | When there is awareness of conflict between reference values (or error) within an individual then the reorganization process begins to make random changes. Trial-and-error changes continue until the error is reduced | A shift in perspective, or "aha moment," during the therapy process (or outside of therapy) could indicate that reorganization has successfully occurred (Gianakis & Carey, 2011). For example, to return to the client in the goal conflict example, once this client becomes aware of the conflict between child and parent selves they could realize one self better fits certain contexts (such as the parent self at work). |

Source: Reproduced with permission from Morris, L., Mansell, W., & McEvoy, P. (2016). The take control course: Conceptual rationale for the development of a transdiagnostic group for common mental health problems. Frontiers in Psychology, 7, 99. doi:10.3389/fpsyg.2016.00099.

Many of you will not be familiar with PCT, although you may have come across some of the theories and understandings that it has influenced. For example, self-regulatory theories, such as that of Carver and Scheier, have been strongly influenced by PCT (Carver & Scheier, 1990, 1998). Other theorists and theories that have been influenced by PCT include Robin Vallacher in his work on action identification and Klaus Grawe in his work on integrating psychological therapies (Grawe, 2007; Vallacher & Wegner, 1987). Furthermore, a number of theorists have used PCT to understand some of the components of CBT that are effective across disorders. For example, Carey (2011) provides an understanding of exposure based on PCT, which is described in more detail in this and later chapters. Other writers have considered how concepts of PCT resonate with other therapeutic approaches, such as essential principles of person centered therapy of: therapist genuineness (therapist is authentic within the therapy relationship), unconditional positive regard (therapist does not disapprove of aspects of client's experience), and empathic understanding (understanding of the individual clients' internal world) (Higginson et al., 2011). These person centred principles are characteristics associated with low therapist interpersonal control and have influenced a range of therapeutic approaches. As is explained in more detail in this chapter, PCT-based interventions emphasize the importance of the client's control, with it being less important that the therapist feels in control particularly in situations where increased therapist control would limit client control.

PCT provides a distinctive set of understandings and these are outlined in this chapter. This chapter is written with healthcare professionals in mind, so it includes clinical examples where possible.

## Living Is Control

PCT is based on the idea that all living beings, including humans, control their perception to ensure their experience is a certain way. This applies to basic things, such as how warm or cold we want to be, through to more complex life goals, such as having a good relationship with a partner (Higginson et al., 2011). One way of thinking about this is that we have a set of "just rights" in our head, "just rights" being representations of how we want the world to be (Carey, 2006). When our experience within the world matches up to our "just rights" then we act to keep things happening this way, but when conditions change and things are no longer "just right," we act to bring things back to the way that we want them to be.

This approach makes PCT highly distinctive. Sometimes other therapies consider control to be a problem; for example, Steven Hayes who developed Acceptance and Commitment Therapy has stated: "control is the problem" (Hayes, 2004, p. 653). Yet, PCT would propose that if we did not control a multitude of things every day, we would become increasingly overwhelmed by our environment—not washing, dressing, talking, traveling, working—all of these are sophisticated processes of control in action. A PCT approach would suggest that we are aware of our attempts at control mainly when we are finding it difficult, whereas most control happens automatically and without thought. It is this kind of automatic flow of control that we are helping clients to try to restore in their lives. Control is implemented through a process known as a negative feedback loop, which is explained in detail in Chapter 2, Session 2, What Blocks Our Control?

## Control Is Managed Over Many Hierarchical Levels

PCT suggests that our goals are organized hierarchically, this means that goals are represented at different levels. Higher level, long-term goals lead to the setting of subgoals that in turn regulate lower level, shorter term goals. For example, a higher level goal of "being a good friend" could lead to the setting of subgoals, such as "to be helpful" and this in turn could lead to the setting of lower level goals, such as "to contact a friend." The theory itself describes in detail eleven different levels in a hierarchy, but the most important principle to be aware of is that for any goal or problem that is being discussed there are likely to be successively higher levels that indicate why this is important, and lower levels that describe how to implement actions to achieve the goal.

## Loss of Control Causes Distress and Conflict Undermines Control

Sometimes we cannot bring things back to the way we want them to be, we cannot get the world to match up to our "just rights" and we can experience loss of control. A number of reviews support a relationship between control and well-being, and between lack of control and psychological distress (e.g., Chorpita & Barlow, 1998; Fitzsimons & Fuller, 2002; Grawe, 2007; Mansell, 2005). It is common that things do not quite go the way that we want them to and this in itself is not the problem. What is suggested to be problematic is when we have important goals that remain in conflict. Carey & Mullan (2008) gives the example of a client, with symptoms of anxiety, who had an on-going conflict between "wanting to let her daughter do normal things" and "wanting to keep her safe." As well as leading to anxiety, these goals informed certain actions at lower levels, which were problematic for the client; for example, trying to stop her daughter going out of the house.

According to Carey, the principle of conflict being at the heart of psychological distress is rather like a theory of "relativity" for psychology. For example, the negative thought "I will make a fool of myself and other people with laugh at me" is only a problem for someone who wants to come across as competent and serious—in other words, it creates conflict (Carey, Mansell, & Tai, 2015). The same thought has an opposite implication for a stand-up comedian or a clown, whose goal is exactly to act foolish and make other people laugh. The same principle can be applied to any behavior or process—it is only a problem if it creates or maintains conflict.

## Conflicts Between Higher Level Goals Cause Greater Problems Than Conflicts at Lower Levels

According to PCT, it is when important, higher level goals remain in conflict that we experience psychological distress and unwanted symptoms. One of the reasons for this is that the higher level goals set the goals for the levels below—they are longer term and more definitional to the self. One way of thinking of this is that the higher level systems that set the conflicted goals are the root of the problem. Without change at the root of the problem, any other changes will not fully address the issue. Although problematic symptoms and behaviors can be highly distressing, they are generally not the "root" of the problem, unless it is these symptoms and behaviors that are blocking awareness of conflicted goals, or conflicting with goals themselves. For example, when people engage in rumination or worry over long periods of time about everyday stresses, this could prevent attention being directed to where the more significant problems lie. On the other hand, targeted worry about an important concern (e.g. recently being attacked in the street) may have a beneficial effect in seeking help or engaging in actions to prevent more serious outcomes.

An example to illustrate the importance of higher level goal conflict is a client who has a higher level conflict between "I need to express how I feel in relationships" and "I must not upset other people." This conflict led to a range of problems because as soon as she thought about telling other people how she felt, she became so concerned that she would upset them that she suppressed the feelings and avoided meeting them. Over time, this led to greater feelings of anger and frustration with other people, and even more avoidance of seeing them. She found that when she tried to force herself to express her feelings, this only led her to feel more guilty and concerned about the impact on other people. So, shifting the lower level goals merely perpetuated the conflict. However, the more she became aware that she was in a conflict between expressing her feelings and not upsetting other people, the more she realized that both sides were a normal part of feeling worthwhile (the overarching goal that drove the conflict) and she needed to change the way she balanced these two goals in different situations. See Fig. 2.1 for a diagrammatic representation of this.

For those who are familiar with a traditional CBT framework, it could be interesting to consider how the concept of higher level goals relates to the concept of core beliefs (Higginson et al., 2011). Certainly, it appears that accessing this level of cognition is of benefit in CBT. However, in contrast, a PCT approach regards "I want to feel worthwhile" as the goal to discuss; the belief of "I am worthless" is merely be the result of long periods of not achieving a feeling of being worthwhile owing to the kinds of conflict we have discussed. Thus, a PCT approach has the capacity to reframe a core belief as the consequence of difficulties with a normal, dynamic, positively orientated goal that can be openly discussed and better understood.

## Control Without Awareness Can Exacerbate Conflict

Within PCT, there is an important role for awareness because without awareness of conflicted goals then conflicts will not be resolved. Lack of awareness of all relevant goals (or reference values) makes it more likely that a goal will be pursued without taking into account another goal that is also controlling this experience. Within PCT, this process of pursuing one goal without taking into account another relevant goal is referred to as *"arbitrary control"* (Powers, 1973).

For example, after a traumatic accident an individual may have recognized the need to discuss their experiences with other people because

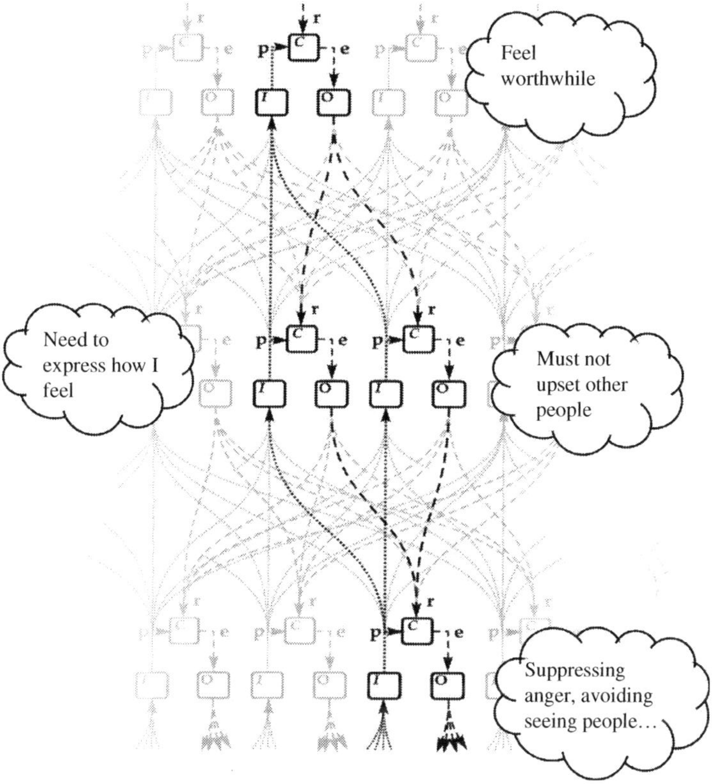


**FIGURE 2.1** Conflict model with a clinical example mapped onto it. Source: *Adapted and reproduced with permission from* A Transdiagnostic Approach to CBT Using Method of Levels Therapy, *by Warren Mansell, Timothy A. Carey, and Sara Tai. Original diagram copyright Dag Forssell.*

they recognize that it will give them support and help them understand how to cope better. However, they might struggle to talk about these experiences due to a second goal they hold, which is to "make sure other people don't think I'm crazy." In practice they may switch between wanting to talk about their problems and wanting to avoid other people. This avoidance then constitutes arbitrary control because they do it despite the impact it has on achieving a goal that is important to them. In PCT, rather than regarding avoidance, or any other "safety seeking behavior", as a problem per se we recognize that it is only a problem to the extent that it causes conflict or keeps it outside awareness. There may be all kinds of benefits to these behaviors as well. Therefore, we help people fully explore the costs and benefits of their behavior, and work out for themselves how to reduce the negative impact they have. Sometimes this might involve gaining better control of when they engage in the behavior and when to not use it.

According to PCT, *arbitrary control* between individuals is a very important to consider because it creates conflict. For example, the criticism of a highly critical friend or family member could interfere with that person's goal of "feeling good about myself." This criticism blocks an important personal goal and so it constitutes arbitrary control. But even what seem to be quite innocuous behaviors on the surface can have the same damaging effects. For example, ignoring a family member when they express their needs, or applying one's own expectations of what is a good achievement to other people. Fig. 2.2 illustrates how arbitrary control maintains the loss of control involved in psychological distress via its effect on blocking important personal goals.

## Change Occurs When Awareness Is Brought to Enduring Higher Level Conflicts, for Long Enough to Allow Their Successful Reorganization

Awareness of conflicted goals is important within a PCT account, as it is suggested that goals cannot change until we have some awareness of them. PCT suggests that changes to our goals occur at the point within the control system at which we are currently aware. The proposed change mechanism within PCT is known as reorganization (Powers, 1973). When there is a loss of control (or error) within the control system then the reorganization process begins to make random

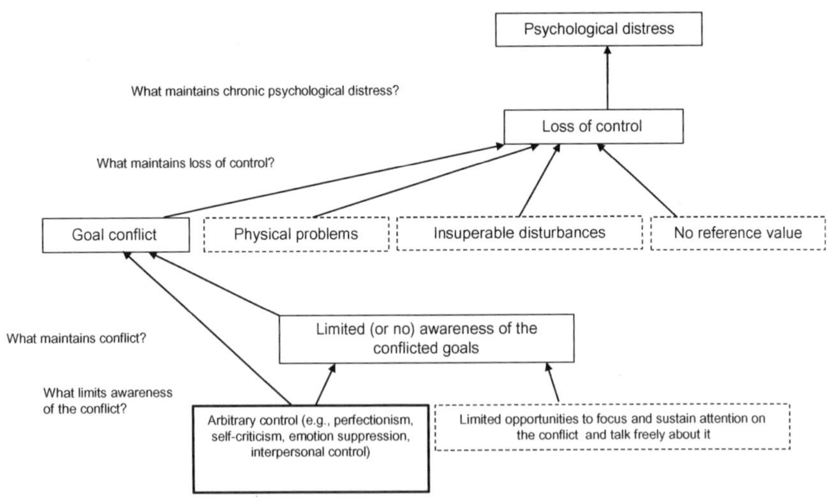


**FIGURE 2.2** A diagram to illustrate how arbitrary control contributes to goal conflict, which in turn contributes to chronic loss of control and psychological distress. Source: *Reproduced with permission from* A Transdiagnostic Approach to CBT Using Method of Levels Therapy, *by Warren Mansell, Timothy A. Carey, and Sara Tai.*

changes (Powers, 1973). Trial-and-error changes in the properties of the control systems continue until loss of control (error) is reduced (Carey, 2011; Powers, 1973). The clinical implications of this include explaining the findings that sudden psychological change (gains, insights, or aha moments) within therapy can result in lasting symptom change because these would be examples of successful reorganization (Aderka, Nickerson, Bøe, & Hofmann, 2012). Reorganization can be experienced as things suddenly making sense, being resolved, or seeing what needs to change, etc.

A vital implication of this for psychological interventions is that awareness must be directed to the higher level goals that are setting the conflicted goals so that these can be reorganized. There are a few ways that this process is facilitated within the TCC. Firstly awareness or mindfulness techniques are used within the Course. From a PCT perspective, the main reason for using awareness techniques is to develop a "window" of awareness that can be brought to bear on the thoughts, feelings, and behaviors involved in conflicted goals. As a result of this emphasis, awareness techniques used in the TCC are shorter than those delivered in some other approaches; for example, Mindfulness Based Cognitive Therapy (Segal, Williams, & Teasdale, 2002).

It is important that awareness is directed to problematic feelings or thoughts in a sustained manner because it can take time for awareness to "settle" on the higher level conflict driving the problem. Awareness of higher level conflict is a precursor for this to be reorganized; however, reorganization is a trial-and-error process and may not always hit on the best solution first. For example, a client may experience a heightening of distress and symptoms before they experience positive change.

Another way in which awareness is directed to the higher level goals that are setting the conflicted goals is through the way that exposure is delivered. Exposure in the TCC is designed to help people hold perceptual conflict in mind and establish a new organization of goals that allows them to regain overall control. An example of a perceptual conflict is between the desire to give a presentation and the fear of looking incompetent, or a conflict between avoiding a past distressing memory and the desire to bring this to mind to make sense of it. So, in the TCC, exposure exercises are client-driven and framed in such a way that they are guided by clients' life goals to promote sustained attention on personally relevant conflicts.

## SUMMARY

This section aims to give a brief overview of key components of PCT, but for more comprehensive accounts of PCT and the evidence base for its components, see Mansell and Carey (2009), Mansell, Carey, and Tai (2012), and Marken and Mansell (2013). Also Morris, Mansell, and McEvoy (2016) give a more detailed summary of PCT and the ways in which PCT has informed the TCC. Box 2.1 provides a summary of key PCT concepts. We are aware that many readers will not be very familiar with PCT so key theoretical points will be revisited as we introduce the material covered in each session. The next chapter provides a brief overview of the TCC and an introduction to the PCT basis of each session.

BOX 2.1

## SUMMARY OF KEY PCT CONCEPTS (INFORMED BY POWERS, 1973 AND MORRIS, MANSELL, & McEVOY, 2016)

1. *Living is control.* PCT is based on the idea that all living beings control their perceptions in order to make their experience a certain way. We all have internal standards, a sense of how we would like our experience to be, and we act on our environment to make our experience match these standards.
2. *Control is managed over many hierarchical levels.* People's goals are organized over a number of different levels. Goals are arranged in a hierarchy with higher level, more general, goals setting the goals for lower levels.
3. *Loss of control causes distress.* When people are unable to control their experiences over a period of time, then they experience distress. Significant loss of control can be a really frightening and disorientating experience and it is not surprising that it can result in a range of distressing symptoms.
4. *Conflict undermines control.* Conflicts will regularly arise between the goals people are trying to achieve; however, when these conflicts are enduring they can result in psychological distress and unwanted symptoms.
5. *Conflicts between higher level goals cause greater problems than conflicts at lower levels.* Chronic conflicts at higher levels result in greater psychological distress than conflicts at lower levels. A specific conflict between "doing a presentation" and "wanting to avoid giving a presentation" does not undermine control to the same extent as a conflict between "being a good employee" and "I can't cope in social situations."

*continued*

**BOX 2.1 (*cont'd*)**

6. *Control without awareness can exacerbate conflict.* If control is applied to an experience in order to meet a goal and does not take into account a competing goal, then one of the goals will be "blocked." This causes conflict as only one of the goals is achieved. For example, one might avoid presentations to prevent anxiety without thinking about how much one wants to present to demonstrate this capability and potentially improve career progression.
7. *Change occurs when awareness is brought to enduring higher level conflicts, for long enough to allow their successful reorganization.* Change occurs through a process called reorganization and reorganization occurs at the point in the hierarchy that the person is aware. Given the importance of higher level goal conflicts within a PCT account, it is vital that awareness is brought to the higher level systems driving the enduring conflict that is creating distress.

# KEY POINTS

- Perceptual Control Theory (PCT) is a transdiagnostic theory that proposes generic mechanisms that account for psychological distress across disorders.
- A key focus is recognizing that we "control" our experiences to make our experiences a certain way.
- Enduring conflicts cause people to perceive that they have lost control and to experience distressing symptoms.

## References

Aderka, I. M., Nickerson, A., Bøe, H. J., & Hofmann, S. G. (2012). Sudden gains during psychological treatments of anxiety and depression: A meta-analysis. *Journal of Consulting and Clinical Psychology, 80*(1), 93. Available from https://doi.org/10.1037/a0026455.

Carey, T. A. (2006). *The method of levels: How to do psychotherapy without getting in the way.* Living Control Hayward, CA, Systems Publishing.

Carey, T. A. (2011). Exposure and reorganization: The what and how of effective psychotherapy. *Clinical Psychology Review, 31*(2), 236–248, [Presents a PCT account of exposure].

Carey, T. A., Mansell, W., & Tai, S. (2015). *Principles-based counselling and psychotherapy: A Method of Levels approach.* London, UK, Routledge.

Carey, T. A., & Mullan, R. J. (2008). Evaluating the method of levels. *Counselling Psychology Quarterly, 21*, 247–256. Available from https://doi.org/10.1080/09515070802396012.

Carver, C. S., & Scheier, M. F. (1990). Origins and functions of positive and negative affect: A control-process view. *Psychological Review*, *97*(1), 19. Available from https://doi.org/10.1037/0033-295X.97.1.19.

Carver, C. S., & Scheier, M. F. (1998). *On the self-regulation of behavior*. Cambridge: Cambridge University Press.

Chorpita, B. F., & Barlow, D. H. (1998). The development of anxiety: The role of control in the early environment. *Psychological Bulletin*, *124*(1), 3. Available from https://doi.org/10.1037/0033-2909.124.1.3.

Fitzsimons, S., & Fuller, R. (2002). Empowerment and its implications for clinical practice in mental health: A review. *Journal of Mental Health*, *11*(5), 481–499. Available from https://doi.org/10.1080/09638230020023.

Grawe, K. (2007). *Neuropsychotherapy: How the neurosciences inform effective psychotherapy*. Mahwah, NJ and London: Lawrence Erlbaum Associates.

Hayes, S. C. (2004). Acceptance and commitment therapy, relational frame theory, and the third wave of behavioral and cognitive therapies. *Behavior Therapy*, *35*(4), 639–665.

Higginson, S., Mansell, W., & Wood, A. M. (2011). An integrative mechanistic account of psychological distress, therapeutic change and recovery: The Perceptual Control Theory approach. *Clinical Psychology Review*, *31*(2), 249–259. Available from https://doi.org/10.1016/j.cpr.2010.01.005, [An overview of PCT and discussion of how concepts within PCT integrate with different psychological approaches].

Mansell, W. (2005). Control theory and psychopathology: An integrative approach. *Psychology and Psychotherapy-Theory Research and Practice*, *78*, 141–178. Available from https://doi.org/10.1348/147608304x21400.

Mansell, W., & Carey, T. A. (2009). A century of psychology and psychotherapy: Is an understanding of 'control' the missing link between theory, research, and practice? *Psychology and Psychotherapy-Theory Research and Practice*, *82*(3), 337–353. Available from https://doi.org/10.1348/147608309x432526.

Mansell, W., Carey, T. A., & Tai, S. J. (2012). *A transdiagnostic approach to CBT using method of levels therapy: distinctive features*. New York: Routledge.

Marken, R. S., & Mansell, W. (2013). Perceptual control as a unifying concept in psychology. *Review of General Psychology*. Available from https://doi.org/10.1037/a0032933.

Morris, L., Mansell, W., & McEvoy, P. (2016). The Take Control Course: Conceptual rationale for the development of a transdiagnostic group for common mental health problems. *Frontiers in Psychology*. Available from https://doi.org/10.3389/fpsyg.2016.00099. Available from http://journal.frontiersin.org/article/10.3389/fpsyg.2016.00099/abstract.

Powers, W. T. (1973). *Behavior: The control of perception*. Chicago, IL: Aldine.

Powers, W. T., Clark, R., & Mc Farland, R. (1960a). A general feedback theory of human behavior: Part I. *Perceptual and Motor Skills*, *11*(1), 71–88. Available from https://doi.org/10.2466/pms.1960.11.1.71.

Powers, W. T., Clark, R., & Mc Farland, R. (1960b). A general feedback theory of human behavior: Part II. *Perceptual and Motor Skills*, *11*(3), 309–323. Available from https://doi.org/10.2466/pms.1960.11.3.309.

Segal, Z. V., Williams, J. M. G., & Teasdale, J. D. (2002). *Mindfulness-based cognitive therapy for depression: A new approach to preventing relapse*. New York and London: Guilford Press.

Vallacher, R. R., & Wegner, D. M. (1987). What do people think they're doing? Action identification and human behavior. *Psychological Review*, *94*(1), 3. Available from https://doi.org/10.1037/0033-295X.94.1.3.

CHAPTER

# 3

# PCT Within Psychological Interventions

Perceptual Control Theory (PCT) provides an account of the causes, and maintenance, of psychological distress. Such an understanding has been applied across a wide variety of presentations, such as phobias (Mansell, 2005), obsessive–compulsive disorder (Pitman, 1987), depression (Hyland, 1987), bipolar disorder (Mansell, 2010), addiction (Webb, Sniehotta, & Michie, 2010), and dissociative disorders (Johnson, 2009; Mansell & Carey, 2012). Although the conflicted goals might be different in each presentation (e.g., facing verses avoiding a specific object in phobia, or conflicting self-states in dissociative identity disorder), the underlying cause of the distress is the same process of prolonged goal conflict outside of awareness. Given the broad application of PCT and both qualitative and quantitative studies providing empirical support, a comprehensive account is not possible here—for a more detailed summary of the evidence for PCT as an account of psychological distress and recovery, see Alsawy, Mansell, Carey, McEvoy, and Tai (2014).

## PERCEPTUAL CONTROL THEORY APPLIED WITHIN INDIVIDUAL INTERVENTIONS

An individual cognitive behavioral therapy (CBT) therapy has been developed based on the principles of PCT. This is called Method of Levels (MOL) (Carey, 2006) and aims to help clients to become aware of higher level goals and facilitate the process of reorganization, in order to resolve goal conflicts (Carey, 2006, 2008). This is achieved by encouraging the client to talk about their problem and by asking about "disruptions." Disruptions can be a smile or a shake of the head, hand gestures, etc. These are important because they indicate a shift in a person's awareness, which could be a shift to higher level thoughts or

*Transdiagnostic Group Therapy Training and Implementation*
DOI: https://doi.org/10.1016/B978-0-12-813989-9.00003-8

understandings of the topic being discussed (Powers, 1998). Curious questions are asked about the problem being discussed and the disruptions in order to direct the client's awareness to their present-moment experience of the problem. An example of such a curious questioning style is provided in Chapter 4, How to Use This Book, as we recommend the use of this questioning style within interactions during the Take Control Course (TCC).

There are manuals available that describe, in detail, the use of PCT in individual therapy. These are included in the further reading list at the end of this chapter.

There have been a number of evaluations of MOL in uncontrolled trials. These have shown significant reductions in symptoms on standardized measures of psychological distress after MOL, with moderate to large effect sizes, for clients experiencing a range of problems including depression, bereavement, anxiety disorders (e.g., social anxiety disorder, posttraumatic stress disorder), relationship breakdowns, and anger management (Carey, 2005; Carey, Carey, Mullan, Spratt, & Spratt, 2009; Carey & Mullan, 2007, 2008). A study of MOL with clients in secondary care calculated an efficiency ratio, which was in order to examine the magnitude of symptom change in relation to the number of sessions attended. As is common in studies of MOL, clients were able to attend the number of sessions that they perceived would be helpful. The improvements demonstrated in this study were of a similar level to other therapies and the efficiency ratio was higher in this study than in all the comparison studies, which included a range of different therapies (Carey, Tai, & Stiles, 2013). This indicates that letting clients choose the sessions that they attend does not make therapy inefficient, and on the contrary this client-led approach makes it more efficient. A pilot Randomized Controlled Trial (RCT) has been conducted in a primary care psychology service (Bird, Tai, Hamilton, & Mansell, 2013) where MOL was compared to control (waiting list or regular CBT treatment). Significant improvements were found on ratings of anxiety and depression in both conditions and there were larger improvements in the MOL condition for ratings of anxiety.

A computerized adaptation of MOL called MYLO (Manage Your Life Online) has been developed. It uses sophisticated searches of words and phrases in clients' typed statements to simulate an MOL-style conversation. In a nonclinical sample, MYLO was associated with a decrease in anxiety, depression, and stress (Gaffney, Mansell, Edwards, & Wright, 2013). A small pilot study ($N = 23$) of a MOL-based app (MindSurf) with nonclinical participants found a nonsignificant decrease in anxiety, depression, and stress scores (Carey, Haviland, Tai, Vanags, & Mansell, 2016). Participants received MOL-style questions on their mobile phones over a 1-week period and reported generally finding the app helpful and convenient (e.g., by enhancing self-awareness and increasing present-moment thinking).

General information and resources regarding applying PCT to mental health problems can be found at: http://www.pctweb.org/psy/mental.html, and the MOL website is http://www.methodoflevels.com.au.

## RESEARCH FOCUSING ON THE TAKE CONTROL COURSE

The effectiveness and feasibility of the TCC was examined in a prospective cohort study comparing TCC with a nonrandomized control group of clients accessing individual low-intensity CBT (LI CBT) (Morris et al., 2016). Individual LI CBT includes guided self-help and other brief clinician-facilitated psychological interventions. The primary outcome was a composite depression and anxiety score. Comparison points were 1-month post baseline (TCC $n = 26$; LI CBT $n = 14$) and 3-months follow-up (TCC $n = 12$; LI CBT $n = 7$). For the TCC group, changes on all pre–post outcomes were significant with moderate effect sizes. The between group effect was not statistically significant; although TCC showed lower mean scores at 1 and 3 months compared to LI CBT (Morris et al., 2016). Also understanding and satisfaction ratings were taken every TCC session ($N = 186$) and the median understanding rating was 9/10 ($IQR = 2.38$) and the median satisfaction rating was 8/10 ($IQR = 3$) However, this study was not a RCT and so there are of sources of bias, e.g., differences between the two treatment groups, which could have influenced the results obtained.

A large single-blind noninferiority RCT ($N = 156$) within Salford (Greater Manchester, UK) compared the TCC to individual LI CBT (Morris, 2016). Primary outcomes (depression and anxiety scores) were measured at 6-month follow-up. Intention-to-treat analyses indicated that TCC was noninferior to individual LI CBT on anxiety and depression outcomes, functioning and an idiosyncratic problem measure. A second, per-protocol analyses found inconclusive evidence of noninferiority. The full dataset (including 12-month follow-up) is currently under analysis. Although this study had a number of strengths including single-blind assessments, prespecified protocol, conservative noninferiority margin, accounting for clustering by group within analyses and combining a RCT design with a naturalistic service setting, there were a number of limitations. These included: the fact that participants were not formally diagnosed and that recruitment was from one specific service covering the specific area of Salford. The per-protocol analysis was limited by the relatively low attendance of treatment sessions across both treatment groups; this is likely to reflect the level of socioeconomic deprivation within the recruitment area (Morris et al., 2016; O'Brien, Fahmy, & Singh, 2009).

A qualitative study of 12 semistructured interviews with individuals who accessed the TCC explored whether the brief transdiagnostic format of the TCC was acceptable and explored participants' perceptions of psychological change (Morris, Mansell, Amos & Edge, 2016). Three superordinate themes were identified: "Style and Format," "Control and Flexibility," and "Change." The results indicated that TCC was acceptable to participants, as satisfaction and understanding levels were generally high. The "Style and Format" theme indicated that participants valued the flexibility of the TCC and generally liked the brief format. Themes regarding "Control and Flexibility" suggested that the theoretical threads of control and awareness were understood and utilized by participants. Furthermore, findings indicated that clarification and awareness of important goals helped participants to understand how they could best meet these goals and "let go" of things they could not control. The majority of participants described a number of changes during the courses, and 10 participants were still using understandings and techniques from the TCC 4–8 months after attending. One of the most striking changes was that six participants described changes in how they related to other people. This was somewhat surprising given that this is not an explicit focus of the TCC, although there is some focus upon this in session 4 and the course is designed to be relevant to a range of participant goals.

## COMPONENTS OF THE TAKE CONTROL COURSE (INCLUDING THE RATIONALE BASED ON PCT)

There is a strong emphasis on client self-direction and control within the TCC, which reflects the evidence base that psychological change (or gains) happen at different time for different people. Also promoting client control as much as possible aims to make it more likely that they are meeting their own goals, rather than being heavily influenced by the clinician's goals. Therefore clients are given information regarding the content of each session and are advised that they do not have to attend a session if they do not think it is relevant. Specific homework tasks are not given, but at the end of each session participants reflect on what they are taking from the session and are encouraged to write down a specific task if relevant. Sessional evaluation forms are filled in and session content can be slightly adapted in response to feedback. Although the core content of each session is prescribed, certain techniques reoccur and so later implementation of techniques can be changed or explained differently in response to feedback. Furthermore, there is an emphasis on experiential learning (trying things out) in order to promote individual clients to consider the relevance, and application, of techniques to themselves.

Each session includes videos of clients who have accessed either previous interventions or earlier TCC. These provide opportunities for the group to hear accounts of other people's experiences of distress and the things that helped them gain more control, as relevant to the session theme. Some opportunities are provided for participants to share their personal experience, but it is strongly emphasized that clients do not have to share these experiences if they do not want to.

In accordance with PCT, targeted throughout the TCC are: (1) understanding the process of control, including the degree to which one can, and desires, control over various aspects of one's life; (2) awareness of valued higher level goals (and reasons for change); (3) awareness of higher level goal conflict; (4) encouragement of flexible ways to control and reduction of processes (including rules, habits, routines, and mental processes) that block valued goals.

The following is a description of key themes of the six sessions with a brief explanation of the PCT rationale. See Appendix B for the list of session themes that we provide to clients (this is also provided on the companion website). If you want a more detailed account of how the PCT basis has informed individual sessions, please see Morris, Mansell and McEvoy (2016). The themes will be revisited when individual sessions are described and more detail will be given then!

*Session 1: "Thinking about control."* Control is the basis of this course. The overall theme in this session is to understand control and to encourage clients to consider the things that they can, and want to, have more control over. Exercises also support clients to consider which of their habits get in the way of them achieving the things that are important to them.

*Session 2: "What blocks our control? Addressing negative thinking: self-critical voice, worry and dwelling on things."* A key message here is that individual thoughts, even negative ones, are not a problem. Even worry, self-criticism, and rumination are normal processes that most people engage in. They are a problem only to the extent that they get in the way of important life goals, or they limit a person's awareness of them. This message is both normalizing and empowering, giving clients the opportunity to think carefully about how and why they do these things, rather than feeling they must stop doing something that has been part of their way of being for many years.

*Session 3: "Feeling in control short-term versus getting control of your life."* The principle of a hierarchy provides a key basis of this session.

A fundamental message of the session is that sometimes our attempts to control our emotions, avoid distress or keep safe can actually get in the way of us doing things that are really important to us. This encourages clients to focus on their longer term (higher-level) goals and to consider how to prioritize these over short-term goals that are getting in the way.

*Session 4: "Taking control of the things around you."* A unique theme of PCT is that we are designed to control our environment for our own purposes. There are many things in our environment that we can change in order to make our world more like we want it to be. However, there are also some things that, objectively, we will have limited control over. Part of our world is other people. This session focuses on helping people take a wider perspective on their own needs and balancing them with those of people who are important to them.

*Session 5: "Building on strengths, qualities, and resources."* The focus of the session is to encourage participants to recall the strengths, qualities, and resources they have, especially at times when things are difficult for them. These are the things inside themselves and within their social world that will help them take control of their lives.

*Session 6: "Moving forward: what gets me stuck? What helps?"* The focus of the session is on consolidating what has been learnt and planning for the future. Clients are encouraged to choose elements of the TCC that they want to revisit. Allowing choice in the material covered, and encouraging clients to reflect on what works for them and when, encourages flexible control. Planning for the future uses what PCT describes as the "imagination mode" and the theory behind this is detailed in Chapter 6, Session 2 What Blocks Our Control?, which is the chapter covering session 6.

*In the next chapter* we will describe how to set up a TCC and go into more detail regarding the overall style of the course.

## KEY POINTS

- Perceptual Control Theory (PCT) has been used effectively to inform psychological interventions.
- An individual therapy called Method of Levels (MOL), based on PCT, has been found to be a useful transdiagnostic intervention.
- PCT-based interventions emphasize key "PCT relevant" themes, such as maximizing client control.

## References

Alsawy, S., Mansell, W., Carey, T. A., McEvoy, P., & Tai, S. J. (2014). Science and practice of transdiagnostic CBT: A Perceptual Control Theory (PCT) Approach. *International Journal of Cognitive Therapy, 7*(4), 334–359. Available from https://doi.org/10.1521/ijct.2014.7.4.334.

Bird, T., Tai, S., Hamilton, A., & Mansell, W. (2013). A pilot randomised controlled trial of method of levels as a transdiagnostic intervention within a primary care psychology service. In *Paper presented at the British Association of Behavioural and Cognitive Psychotherapies Annual Conference,* Imperial College, London.

Carey, T. A. (2005). Can patients specify treatment parameters? A preliminary investigation. *Clinical Psychology & Psychotherapy, 12*(4), 326–335. Available from https://doi.org/10.1002/cpp.455.

Carey, T. A. (2006). *The method of levels: How to do psychotherapy without getting in the way.* Hayward: Living Control Systems Publ.

Carey, T. A. (2008). Perceptual Control Theory and the Method of Levels: Further contributions to a transdiagnostic perspective. *International Journal of Cognitive Therapy, 1*(3), 237–255. Available from https://doi.org/10.1521/ijct.2008.1.3.237.

Carey, T. A., Carey, M., Mullan, R. J., Spratt, C. G., & Spratt, M. B. (2009). Assessing the statistical and personal significance of the method of levels. *Behavioural and Cognitive Psychotherapy, 37*(3), 311–324. Available from https://doi.org/10.1017/s1352465809005232.

Carey, T. A., Haviland, J., Tai, S. J., Vanags, T., & Mansell, W. (2016). MindSurf: a pilot study to assess the usability and acceptability of a smartphone app designed to promote contentment, wellbeing, and goal achievement. *BMC psychiatry, 16*(1), 442.

Carey, T. A., & Mullan, R. J. (2007). Patients taking the lead. A naturalistic investigation of a patient led approach to treatment in primary care. *Counselling Psychology Quarterly, 20*(1), 27–40. Available from https://doi.org/10.1080/09515070701211304.

Carey, T. A., & Mullan, R. J. (2008). Evaluating the method of levels. *Counselling Psychology Quarterly, 21*(3), 247–256. Available from https://doi.org/10.1080/09515070802396012.

Carey, T. A., Tai, S. J., & Stiles, W. B. (2013). Effective and efficient: Using patient-led appointment scheduling in routine mental health practice in remote Australia. *Professional Psychology: Research and Practice, 44*(6), 405. Available from https://doi.org/10.1037/a0035038.

Gaffney, H., Mansell, W., Edwards, R., & Wright, J. (2013). Manage Your Life Online (MYLO): A pilot trial of a conversational computer-based intervention for problem solving in a student sample. *Behavioural and Cognitive Psychotherapy,* 1–16. Available from https://doi.org/10.1017/S135246581300060X.

<http://www.methodoflevels.com.au>.

Hyland, M. E. (1987). Control theory interpretation of psychological mechanisms of depression: Comparison and integration of several theories. *Psychological Bulletin, 102* (1), 109–121. Available from https://doi.org/10.1037/0033-2909.102.1.109.

Johnson, R. (2009). The intrapersonal civil war. *Psychologist, 22*(4), 300.

Mansell, W. (2005). Control theory and psychopathology: An integrative approach. *Psychology and psychotherapy-Theory research and practice, 78,* 141–178. Available from https://doi.org/10.1348/147608304x21400.

Mansell, W. (2010). Bipolar Disorders. In A. Grant, M. Townend, R. Mulhern, & N. Short (Eds.), *Cognitive behaviour therapy in mental health care (2nd ed.).* London: SAGE Publications Ltd.

Mansell, W., & Carey, T. (2012). Dissociation: Perceptual control theory as an integrative framework for clinical interventions. In F. Kennedy, H. Kennerly, & D. Pearson (Eds.), *Cognitive behavioural approaches to the understanding and treatment of dissociation* (pp. 221–235). London: Routledge.

Morris, L. (2016). *Examination of the effectiveness and acceptability of a transdiagnostic group for clients with common mental health problems* (Unpublished doctoral thesis). Manchester: University of Manchester.

Morris, L., Mansell, W., Amos, R., & Edge, D. (2016). Experiences of a transdiagnostic group, the Take Control Course, for clients with common mental health problems: a qualitative study. Manuscript submitted for publication.

Morris, L., Mansell, W., Emsley, R., Bates, R., Comiskey, J., Pistorius, E., & McEvoy, P. (2016). Prospective cohort feasibility study of a transdiagnostic group intervention for common mental health problems: The Take Control Course. *Psychology and Psychotherapy: Theory, Research and Practice, 89*(2), 163–180.

Morris, L., Mansell, W., & McEvoy, P. (2016). The Take Control Course: Conceptual rationale for the development of a transdiagnostic group for common mental health problems. *Frontiers in Psychology*. Available from https://doi.org/10.3389/fpsyg.2016.00099.

O'Brien, A., Fahmy, R., & Singh, S. P. (2009). Disengagement from mental health services. *Social Psychiatry and Psychiatric Epidemiology, 44*(7), 558–568. Available from https://doi.org/10.1007/s00127-008-0476-0.

Pitman, R. K. (1987). A cybernetic model of obsessive-compulsive psychopathology. *Comprehensive Psychiatry, 28*(4), 334–343. Available from https://doi.org/10.1016/0010-440X(87)90070-8.

Powers, W. T. (1998). *Making sense of behavior: the meaning of control*. New Canaan, CT: Benchmark Publications.

<http://www.pctweb.org/psy/mental.html>.

Webb, T. L., Sniehotta, F. F., & Michie, S. (2010). Using theories of behaviour change to inform interventions for addictive behaviours. *Addiction, 105*(11), 1879–1892. Available from https://doi.org/10.1111/j.1360-0443.2010.03028.x.

## Further Reading

Therapy manuals for PCT in individual therapy:

Carey, T. (2008). *Hold that thought! Two steps to effective counseling and psychotherapy with the Method of Levels*. Chapel Hill, NC: New View Publishing.

Mansell, W., Carey, T. A., & Tai, S. J. (2012). *A Transdiagnostic Approach to CBT Using Method of Levels Therapy: Distinctive Features*. New York: Routledge.

CHAPTER

# 4

# How to Use This Book

In this chapter, we will give an overview of how to make use of this book. We will summarize the client groups that it is most likely to be helpful for. We will then give an overview of the Take Control Course (TCC) and the material in this book, including the overall format of the course and how to set up and organize courses.

## WHO IS THE TAKE CONTROL COURSE FOR?

The TCC is a transdiagnostic intervention. This means that it is aimed at clients with a range of problems, including symptoms of anxiety and depression (see Chapter 1, Introduction to This Book and the Take Control Course, and Chapter 2, Conceptual and Theoretical Background, for more details regarding transdiagnostic approaches). Although the TCC is a transdiagnostic, the format of the TCC is fairly brief (six sessions). Therefore the research so far has looked at how effective it is in primary care services as there is a stronger evidence base for brief interventions within such services (e.g., Richards & Borglin, 2011). We expect that the course will be relevant to a much wider range of clients, but there may need to be adaptations, and regular monitoring and feedback from clients, to ensure that the TCC is meeting their needs; see Part C, Chapter 13, Taking Practice Forward, for more discussion of this (Morris, Mansell, & McEvoy, 2016). Consequently, if you are interested in providing the course beyond primary care, we would encourage you to contact us and work together on adapting it.

Like any psychological intervention the TCC should be offered to clients on the basis of their goals and preferences. For example, if a client specifically wants to "talk things over" in some detail then the TCC is unlikely to be the best option for them. Similarly, if a client really does not want to access an intervention delivered in a course format then the TCC is not going to be the best option. While always

*Transdiagnostic Group Therapy Training and Implementation*
DOI: https://doi.org/10.1016/B978-0-12-813989-9.00004-X

being sure to respect clients' wishes, it is often worth ensuring that clients are clear about what the format of the TCC is. It can be helpful to explicitly say that the course is not at all like the stereotype of Alcoholics Anonymous (AA) meetings, where everyone gets up and talks about their problems! This is not done to persuade clients that they should attend the course if they do not want to, but to help make sure that they do not miss out because they think it is something it is not.

It is also possible that some clients might need an alternative approach or more than one psychological intervention. Again, this is common to all psychological interventions and cannot be entirely prevented even though the use of careful clinical assessment.

## USING THIS BOOK

### Structure of the Book

This book is laid out so that every chapter (after this one) describes a single session of the TCC. The full TCC is six sessions; the first session is an hour and a quarter, and the other five sessions are 1-h each. As well as describing the session, relevant theoretical points will be briefly covered—we are aware that PCT will be new to some people!

Worksheets are included for each session on the companion website. The extra worksheets that we give people at the end of certain sessions are also included on the companion website.

### Session "Overviews"

Each chapter includes an overview of the components of the relevant session. A summary of these is provided in a format that is easy to print out and use during the session. The summaries that can be printed out for use in the session are called "facilitator session guides" and are included in Appendix E and on the companion website. Although some of the overviews contain scripts of what to say, we do not expect these to be learnt by heart. They are provided to give a clear illustration of the kind of language and explanation used. Facilitators will have different styles, and as you become more familiar with the material, it is likely that you will adapt the style and language used to suit your style and the group that you are addressing.

### Using a Perceptual Control Theory Style

The theoretical understanding of perceptual control theory (PCT; Powers, 1973) is critical to the style of delivery. The aim is to encourage clients to control in the broadest sense. Recall that effective control is driven by people's higher level goals—i.e., their ideals, values, and long-term aspirations. The facilitator of the group is therefore aware that there will always be reasons behind any question asked, and behind any particular behavior that a person engages in. They may not be aware of these or their impact at the time. Arbitrary control is the opposite of this overarching control because it does not take into account all of a client's important goals. Therefore the kind of flexible control that is promoted takes into account all of a client's important goals and how these are related. One important implication of this is that a behavior is only seen as a problem if it is incompatible with achieving another goal that is important to the client. For example, worry would only be a problem if it conflicts with another important goal, such as "having a happy life" or "resolving my current problems."

Another important implication, which follows on from the worry example, is that it is really important for the clinician to encourage a client to make sense of whether a behavior is problematic for them: is it always problematic? Would it still be problematic if they did it less? It is important not to assume that a particular behavior (or cognitive process) is automatically problematic, but to check this out or encourage clients to check this out. Many behaviors and cognitive processes that characterize psychological disorders are also common in the general population; for example, worry and intrusive thoughts have been found to be common (e.g., Eriksen, Svendsrod, Ursin, & Ursin, 1998; Fullana et al., 2009). Such processes can be highly problematic for some people, but the important thing is not to assume.

Overall, each client is treated as a unique individual with their own goals, values, and beliefs, which are respected. The problems that the client describes are seen as a potentially understandable consequence of the kind of life that the client is experiencing, and the challenges inherent in managing conflicting values, beliefs, and goals.

## Curious Questioning Style

This style of "not assuming" leads to a curious questioning style, which is directed toward an understanding of a client's present moment experience and the personal meaning of what they are raising. For example, such a questioning style may be used to develop and understand comments or questions within the group. Clearly it is important to tailor the response to the question asked, if a client asked a very factual question (e.g., when does the session finish) it is unlikely to be appropriate to ask them in detail about their present moment experience! Also given the group context, it is important to be sensitive to what and how much you ask people as it is not an individual therapy session and individuals will vary as to how comfortable they feel sharing with a group. Facilitators could check with clients whether they are comfortable to be asked some questions; for example, "is it OK if I ask you a few questions about that?" An example of a curious questioning style is given in Box 4.1; in this example the client leads the dialogue by asking the facilitator questions. However, the facilitator could still check out with the client whether they are feeling comfortable with the dialogue; for example, "is it OK for you to talk about this now?" or "how is it going talking about this?" This is especially important if the facilitator picks up any cues that the client is uncomfortable, such as reduced eye-contact, slow responses, but it is useful to check even if there are no visible cues of discomfort.

As mentioned, the focus of this questioning style is to encourage clients to elaborate problems and concerns that they are experiencing and the personal significance of these. Ultimately, focusing on personally salient aspects of the conversation facilitates clients to bring awareness to conflicts and deeper values or higher level goals. For example the facilitator may ask about words that seen to have a particular salience, or emotional charge, for the client, such as "normal" in the example Box 4.1. The facilitator may also ask the client "does that bother you?" or "why is that important to you?" to clarify the meaning of events, behaviors, and experiences for the individual client. Questions such as these are an important part of "not assuming." This style of questioning can constitute a therapeutic intervention in itself and has been termed empathic curiosity (McEvoy, Baker, Plant, Hylton, & Mansell, 2013; McEvoy & Plant, 2014). The established intervention based on this sort of questioning style is called method of levels (MOL). A much more detailed account of "PCT-style" questioning and MOL is provided in Mansell, Carey, and Tai (2012).

For those clinicians who familiar with cognitive behavioral therapy, this questioning style has some similarities to Socratic Questioning as described by some leading writers (e.g., Padesky, 1993). However, summarizing or interpretative questioning is not common in a "PCT-style" of questioning. Also, questions are focused particularly around the present moment.

## Evaluation Form (Provided in Appendix C, Sessional Evaluation Form)

A one-page evaluation form has been developed and should be handed out at the end of every session. This should be completed anonymously as the purpose is to get honest feedback on what elements of

## BOX 4.1

## AN EXAMPLE OF AN EXCHANGE USING A CURIOUS QUESTIONING STYLE

| | |
|---|---|
| Client: | Is it normal to think about things over and over again? |
| Clinician: | What does normal mean to you? |
| Client: | Like does everyone think over and over about certain things? Is it healthy to do this? |
| Clinician: | Can I just check with you—you mentioned both "normal" and "healthy" there. Would you say normal and healthy are the same or different? |
| Client: | Different |
| Clinician: | Is one more important to you? |
| Client: | I think being healthy is more important because different people do all kinds of different things. I suppose I'm worried that it is not healthy to keep thinking about things |
| Clinician: | And what do you have in mind when you say "healthy"? |
| Client: | Well, physically OK—not damaging myself |
| Clinician: | So, are you concerned you're damaging yourself? |
| Client: | Yes by dwelling on things and making myself feel bad |
| Clinician: | OK, so would it make sense for you if we do some work in this session on describing the bad things about dwelling too much, but also may be look at what people get out of dwelling on things too? |

The clinician would have a number of options as to how they wanted to further respond to this and this would depend on client preference, where they were up to with the sessions, the potential relevance to other clients, and previous feedback from the group. They might continue the discussion, or bring some psychoeducative materials to the next session, or offer the client opportunity to discuss this with them after the session, or refer to a relevant section of the materials covered in more detail, etc.! Given the format of the sessions, it is always necessary to balance individual and group discussion with covering the core components; for example, some groups will feedback that they find the opportunity to explore and ask questions particularly helpful, but others will feedback that they would prefer to focus on the worksheets and core session components.

the session clients are finding helpful or less helpful. Although people will give verbal feedback, the evaluation form gives everyone the opportunity to express their perspective. A slightly longer version of the evaluation form has been created for the final session; this is provided in Appendix C, and both the sessional and final evaluation forms are also provided on the companion website.

In line with the focus on maximizing client's flexible control, the responses to the evaluation form should be used to inform the next session. Although the core content of each session is prescribed, certain techniques reoccur and so later implementation of techniques can be changed or explained differently in response to feedback. It is necessary to be pragmatic in response to feedback; for example, if one person does not respond to a certain exercise but everyone else really likes the exercise then you would not want to totally remove that element. However, what you could do is explain the exercise in a different way or even acknowledge that the anonymous evaluation forms have indicated that someone is not finding a particular aspect very helpful and giving them the opportunity to discuss this at the end of the session.

## Stories and Metaphors

While explaining certain techniques and ways of understanding, we use stories and metaphors. This is to make the material more engaging and because sometimes a story can be much easier to remember than a load of concepts! We suggest you to explain this at some point, just to make clear why you are delivering some of the material in this way. However, we have not had substantial negative feedback about the use of stories and metaphors, and some people have said how much they like this element.

Imagery and metaphor have been found to be useful intervention components (Holmes, Arntz, & Smucker, 2007; Holmes & Mathews, 2010; Ng, Krans, & Holmes, 2013). A useful resource is the Oxford Guide to metaphors as this gives examples of metaphors in many different contexts (Stott, Mansell, Salkovskis, & Lavender, 2010). This book goes some way to explain the function and mechanism of metaphors, drawing on PCT.

## Handouts

There are handouts for each session. You may photocopy these to give to group members. The main session worksheets are included in each chapter, and supplementary sheets (which are given to clients at the end of some sessions) are included in the appendices. Most of the handouts are the ones that clients will be asked to complete during the session, this follows on from the emphasis on trying out techniques, and ways of thinking about things, to encourage flexible control. Some slides and session sheets are described as "reference," this is used when the slide or sheet is provided for a visual reference but clients do not need to refer to or complete these.

### PowerPoint Slides

There are slides for each session. These include the videos of previous clients' experiences. The slides containing client videos are available on the companion website for this book.

### Condensed Session Sheets and Session Guides

Condensed session sheets and session guides are provided for each session. The condensed session sheets provide a brief overview of what will be covered in the sessions. The session guides provide more detail; they list the main session components and provide a summary of the key points. The session guides can be useful for newer facilitators as they provide prompts as to key utterances and actions. The session guides can also be used to note which facilitator is taking a lead on which section.

## HOW TO ORGANIZE A COURSE

### Room Layout

We arrange the room a bit like a classroom, i.e., with desks in rows and people sitting at the desks. This is to emphasize that the TCC is not a group that focuses on self-disclosure and also to provide clients with some privacy when they are filling in worksheets. At the front there is a projector screen, and the facilitators will stand or sit at the front during most of the exercises. It can be helpful to put the relevant worksheets out on tables, or by the door so that people can pick them up as they come in.

### Facilitator Roles

Courses generally run with two facilitators. It is possible to run a session with one person, e.g., if one facilitator is off, but generally it is better to have two facilitators. Having two facilitators generally means that the group will get the best experience and it is helpful for the facilitators also! For example, one facilitator can be delivering material while the other can keep an eye on whether anyone in the group looks like they are not following the material or seems upset, etc. Also facilitators can support each other by providing examples or clarification of sections that have not been presented clearly.

We would suggest that you agree before the session who is doing what (see "Preparation for the sessions" section) and would generally divide up the material fairly evenly. Generally, we are guided by facilitator preference in dividing up the material; if someone particularly wants to introduce a certain section then we had encourage them to do so.

## Preparation for the Sessions: Each Week

Before each session you will need to meet with your cofacilitator to discuss who is doing what during the next session. Ideally, this is done a few days to a week before the next session to allow you to spend time to practice any aspects that you feel you need to work on. You will also need to agree who is preparing what, e.g., who is printing out the session worksheets for the session.

## Group Processes

This section offers some general pointers regarding working with groups and different group dynamics. The same general stance, described previously, applies in dealing with different interpersonal interactions, which is that each client is treated as a unique individual with their own goals, values, and beliefs. Given that the group consists of a number of different individuals then these varied individuals need to be taken into account.

*Responding to different opinions*. If what the person is saying is not overtly offensive to anyone in the group (e.g., racist comments), explore what they are saying. You can thank them for their opinion/honesty. If someone continues to express the opinion to the extent that it is affecting others in the group then move on; for example, agree to differ. If comments are offensive then please follow the relevant service policy as offensive comments are not appropriate.

*Refocusing*. This may be necessary if you feel the discussion has gone off track. We want to be responsive to group members; however, each individual is not the only person in the group and people will often get frustrated/disinterested if they feel one person is dominating the group.

Try to relate what is being discussed to themes/content of group. If you feel that you need to move on, use phrases like: "thank you for sharing that with, we are going to need to move on or there won't be enough time to cover everything." "We're going to need to move on now but I'm interested in what you are saying, you can talk to me after the session if you want to."

*Dealing with distress.* If the client gets very distressed, panicky, etc., you can normalize the response; allow other group members to support. Do not ignore it or explore it too deeply. Give the person the option to leave the room with one of the facilitators. Find a private space and allow them what they need to feel they want to return to group. Usually, it makes most sense for whoever is less involved in leading the section to go out. Again the emphasis is on checking out what is best for the individual and enabling them to maintain control. Although many facilitators will also be trained clinicians, supporting distressed clients in this context will be different from a therapy session. For example the emphasis is more on supporting the client through this particular experience than on providing a discrete psychological intervention (at times there may be some overlap).

## Equipment

Different rooms have very different facilities. It is important to check what facilities are on offer; for example, do they have a projector, or computer that could connect to a projector, which you could use? If you are using a computer that does not belong to the service, it is important to check for potential issues *before the first group session*, such as the presentations not being compatible with the system or the videos not playing. It is worth checking how loud the videos are in advance and bringing speakers if they are too quiet.

Below are the materials for every session; these are also listed prior to the session plan for each individual session. Facilitators may find it easier to have a bag/other storage item, in which they can keep the materials that are needed repeatedly, e.g., pens, post it notes. It can also be useful to have a file(s) to keep the worksheets and clinical measures organized.

## Materials Required for Every Session

Projector to show PowerPoint
Laptop or computer (to use with projector)
Speakers
USB containing PowerPoint slides
Pens
Clipboards
Spares of previous session worksheets
Evaluation form

Clinical measures: e.g., measures of depression, anxiety, and functioning (PHQ9, GAD7, WSAS, etc.)
Session plans and materials
Record of attendance

## Adherence Rating

Although rating adherence is not compulsory, it can be helpful to establish if there are any areas of facilitation that can be improved. The checklist can be used by each facilitator to self-rate their own performance, or it can be used by an observer or cofacilitator to other rate.

The *Adherence checklist* was developed for use in the initial effectiveness, feasibility, and acceptability study of the TCC and is partly based on Cognitive Therapy Scale-Revised (CTS-R; Blackburn et al., 2001). The manual should be used to inform ratings that made using the *Adherence checklist* as it describes the content of the intervention and the underlying theoretical stance in more detail than was possible for the checklist itself. The checklist and more detail on the items included can be found in Appendix D, Take Control Course: Competence and Adherence Scale.

*In the next chapter*, we will describe the first session.

## KEY POINTS

- TCC is a transdiagnostic intervention.
- An understanding of PCT is essential to the style of delivery.
- It is important that facilitators do not assume that a particular behavior (or cognitive process) is automatically problematic. A curious questioning style helps with this.
- When responding to the group, it is important to check out what is best for individual group members and enable them to maintain control.

## References

Blackburn, I.-M., James, I. A., Milne, D. L., Baker, C., Standart, S., Garland, A., & Reichelt, F. K. (2001). The revised cognitive therapy scale (CTS-R): Psychometric properties. *Behavioural and Cognitive psychotherapy, 29*(04), 431–446.

Eriksen, H. R., Svendsrod, R., Ursin, G., & Ursin, H. (1998). Prevalence of subjective health complaints in the Nordic European countries in 1993. *The European Journal of Public Health, 8*(4), 294–298.

Fullana, M., Mataix-Cols, D., Caspi, A., Harrington, H., Grisham, J., Moffitt, T., & Poulton, R. (2009). Obsessions and compulsions in the community: Prevalence, interference, help-seeking, developmental stability, and co-occurring psychiatric conditions. *American Journal of Psychiatry, 166*(3), 329–336.

Holmes, E. A., Arntz, A., & Smucker, M. R. (2007). Imagery rescripting in cognitive behaviour therapy: Images, treatment techniques and outcomes. *Journal of Behavior Therapy and Experimental Psychiatry, 38*(4), 297–305. Available from https://doi.org/10.1016/j.jbtep.2007.10.007.

Holmes, E. A., & Mathews, A. (2010). Mental imagery in emotion and emotional disorders. *Clinical Psychology Review, 30*(3), 349–362. Available from https://doi.org/10.1012/j.cpr.2010.01.001.

Mansell, W., Carey, T. A., & Tai, S. J. (2012). *A transdiagnostic approach to CBT using method of levels therapy: Distinctive features.* New York: Routledge.

McEvoy, P., Baker, D., Plant, R., Hylton, K., & Mansell, W. (2013). Empathic curiosity: Resolving goal conflicts that generate emotional distress. *Journal of Psychiatric and Mental Health Nursing, 20*(3), 273–278.

McEvoy, P., & Plant, R. (2014). Dementia care: Using empathic curiosity to establish the common ground that is necessary for meaningful communication. *Journal of Psychiatric and Mental Health Nursing, 21*(6), 477–482.

Morris, L., Mansell, W., & McEvoy, P. (2016). The Take Control Course: Conceptual rationale for the development of a transdiagnostic group for common mental health problems. *Frontiers in Psychology, 7*, 99. Available from https://doi.org/10.3389/fpsyg.2016.00099.

Ng, R. M., Krans, J., & Holmes, E. A. (2013). *Mental imagery and psychopathology: Examples of post-traumatic stress disorder and bipolar disorder. Multisensory Imagery* (pp. 365–384). Berlin: Springer.

Padesky, 1993. http://padesky.com/newpad/wp-content/uploads/2012/11/socquest.pd

Powers, W. T. (1973). Behavior: the Control of Perception. Chicago, Il: Aldine.

Richards, D. A., & Borglin, G. (2011). Implementation of psychological therapies for anxiety and depression in routine practice: Two year prospective cohort study. *Journal of Affective Disorders, 133*(1), 51–60. Available from https://doi.org/10.1016/j.jad.2011.03.024.

Stott, R., Mansell, W., Salkovskis, P., & Lavender, A. (2010). *Oxford guide to metaphors in CBT: Building cognitive bridges.* Oxford: Oxford University Press.

# PART B

CHAPTER

# 5

# Session 1 Thinking About Control

## OVERVIEW

In this session we welcome participants to the Course and introduce the key elements of the course. This session also introduces a number of components that come up throughout the course, and so it is more comprehensive that later chapters. Although we encourage Take Control Course (TCC) participants to choose which sessions they want to attend, we advise everyone to attend this first session.

The first part of the chapter details the overall theoretical basis of the session and key session sections. Then each session section is detailed, including the materials required for each section. A list of all the materials for the whole session is provided after the session sections. A condensed session plan is provided after the list of all the session materials. A longer "condensed session plan" is provided in Appendix E and on our companion website. This could be particularly useful for newer facilitators as it provides detail about the different session components in an overview format. This is described as a "facilitator session guide" and there is a session guide for all the sessions in Appendix E (on the first page of Appendix E there is a key to the session guides that details what the italicism, bolding, etc. represents).

## KEY SESSION FOCUS

The overall theme in this session is to understand control and to encourage clients to consider the things that they can, and want to, have more control over. Exercises also support clients to consider which of

*Transdiagnostic Group Therapy Training and Implementation*
DOI: https://doi.org/10.1016/B978-0-12-813989-9.00005-1

their ways of coping get in the way of them achieving the things that are important to them

## OVERALL RATIONALE

The key message of this session is that it is normal to try to control aspects of our lives—in fact, to live is to control. We are often unaware of how many things in our lives we control quite naturally. Yet, many clients are fully aware of the fact that they have lost control over aspects of their lives since their mental health difficulties began. They may well see this as an all-or-nothing change—that they no longer have control over their lives. Therefore, this session includes various methods to help people understand that control is relative, even for the simplest experience. For example, we cannot control whether it is going to rain outside, but we can control how much we get wet—by carrying an umbrella. Similarly, one might not be able to control whether a family member is being critical, but one can control how much one listens to this criticism.

The Perceptual Control Theory (PCT) focus of the session also ensures that the facilitators are interested in what experiences or perceptions are being controlled *by* behavior. When clients are perplexed by their actions, or those of other people, PCT can help illuminate a reason for the behavior. This in itself can be very normalizing. For example, anxious clients may report tensing their muscles. Simple questioning can reveal that this is an attempt to feel less shaky and therefore less anxious. Depressed clients may isolate themselves from other people, and yet criticize themselves for doing so. Questioning often reveals that social withdrawal serves to try to keep them away from people who they think might criticize or reject them. This makes their own behavior more understandable and acceptable. According to PCT, every behavior has a purpose—often one that rings true with the client. This is the case whether or not it achieves that purpose successfully, or leads to other difficulties.

Sometimes, facilitators and clients may struggle with the term "control" because they see it as a bad thing. For example, a "control freak" is a term commonly used to describe someone who tries to dictate to others how everything should be done. A control freak may be regarded as "rigid" or "inflexible" in the standards they set for other people. In turn, other people may become frustrated with them and either refuse to do what the control freak says, or oblige and yet resent the infringement on their freedom.

From the perspective of PCT, someone who is called a "control freak" is clearly not controlling effectively, for the very reasons that we see above—they create conflict with other people through their inflexible ways of applying control. According to PCT, we ultimately control *our own perceptions;* we can attempt to manipulate other people to do this (e.g., "if other people do what I say it means I am a worthwhile person"), but it can be met with conflict when other people's goals are not considered. This is called arbitrary control (Powers, 1973) and it ultimately reduces control because of the conflict it causes. Thus, in the session, if people suggest that control is a problem, the facilitator will ask curious questions to elucidate what they mean, considering that conflict is likely to lurk round the corner when control is not working effectively. See Box 5.1 for an example.

BOX 5.1

## AN EXAMPLE OF AN EXCHANGE USING A CURIOUS QUESTIONING STYLE.

| | |
|---|---|
| Client: | I'm not sure about being controlling. I picture my ex-husband screaming at our daughter. |
| Clinician: | Can I just check—what does being controlling mean to you? |
| Client: | Well, I don't want to be like my ex-husband. He was really controlling. He wanted too much control. |
| Clinician: | Would you say that "control" and being controlling are the same or different? |
| Client: | They are a bit different I suppose. When I'm being controlling I tend to yell at my daughter and go on at her about needing to get a job. |
| Clinician: | And what is it like when you're "in control"? |
| Client: | I don't think I am in control that much, it's like I'm either controlling or other people are controlling me. |
| Clinician: | How does that work for you? |
| Client: | Its rubbish—when I'm controlling I really upset everyone and when other people control me I feel really down and can't be bothered to do anything. |
| Clinician: | How far apart are being controlling and being controlled by others? |
| Client: | They seem miles apart. |
| Clinician: | Is there anything in the middle? |
| Client: | I think that being in control is in the middle, but I don't really know what that looks like. |

*continued*

BOX 5.1 (*cont'd*)

The clinician would have a number of options as to how they wanted to further respond to this. They can ask themselves: how relevant the discussion could be to others in the group? Whether there is a section that could be missed to allow for more discussion? Whether they could link it into the session theme or components covered within the session? For example, Session 4 discusses being "in control" with other people and looks at being assertive as a midpoint between "being controlled" or "being controlling."

As discussed in Chapter 4, How to Use This Book, Part A, it is always necessary to balance individual and group discussion with covering the core components. The evaluation forms and verbal feedback are really useful in understanding what the group is finding most helpful.

Throughout the descriptions of how to deliver the sessions, examples are given of curious questions. These questions are given in order to give readers a sense of the sort of questions that are commonly asked, but facilitators will need to respond appropriately to the flow of discussion and client's individual situations.

This session demonstrates conflict in more detail through exercises and discussion. It is important to note that clients may not use the word "conflict" explicitly. Clients may describe the experience of conflict in more subtle and idiosyncratic ways. For example, they may describe having problems with another person, they may experience "being stuck," being in "two minds" about something, or having "two sides within themselves."

## PCT Rationale for the Brief Awareness Technique and Imaginal Goal-Focused Exposure

PCT proposes that problematic conflict is maintained by a lack of awareness of one of the goals that is causing the conflict. An example may illustrate this. Sarah had a goal of "being independent" and another goal, which she was unaware of, of "being cared for by others." Partly in order to fulfill her goal of being independent she became a very successful business woman, yet at the same time her need for being cared for became more distant. She felt increasingly isolated and low, but could not quite put her finger on why. Sarah's example illustrates how conflict can remain implicit, continuing to contribute to problems, until it is brought into awareness.

PCT suggests that changes to our goals occur at the point within the control system at which we are currently aware. Therefore, bringing awareness to problematic conflicts is really important. The proposed change mechanism within PCT is known as reorganization (Powers, 1973). It is a fundamental process of learning common to all living organisms and so it operates directly on what we are currently perceiving—it is not a logical or intellectual process. This may explain why effective exposure is commonly described as "experiential," i.e., learning through experience. When there is a loss of control (or error) within the control system then the reorganization process begins to make random changes at the point in the system where awareness is focused (Powers, 1973). If the changes result in reducing the error, then these changes will persist. If these changes do not reduce the error, then another change is generated (Powers, 1973). Because reorganization is a trial-and-error process and therefore the first changes may not resolve the problem, it takes a period of time to begin to work. This may explain why successful exposure is sustained on an experience for a period of time.

If you are reading about PCT for the first time, it may well feel as if you are still "getting to grips" with this understanding of how change works. You may have noticed the implications of such a process in clinical practice; for example, change that happens suddenly, but is still significant and lasting. Or initial changes that do not seem like the most helpful ones (due to the random nature of the process)—e.g., sudden strong outbursts of anger as someone tries to be more assertive.

You may also remember from Chapter 2, Conceptual and Theoretical Background, Part A, the importance of reorganization occurring at the "root" of the conflict. We gave the example of a client, called Gemma, who has a higher level goal conflict between "I need to express how I feel in relationships" and "I must not upset other people." She suppressed feelings of anger and dissatisfaction with others and avoided meeting them. She found that when she tried to force herself to express her feelings, this only led her to feel more guilty and concerned about the impact on other people. So, shifting the lower level goals merely perpetuated the conflict. It was only when Gemma became aware of the "root" conflict that she realized that both sides were a normal part of feeling worthwhile. For reorganization to occur at the "root" of conflict, awareness has to be directed there. This may explain why exposure in psychological therapy is carried out within the context of client goals, even though this may not be explicit. For example, the graded hierarchy would be used to help the client move towards something they need or want to face. Generally clinicians would also spend time discussing the value of the exposure process, as "moving towards" a feared or avoided experience is often not immediately appealing. This might often involve discussing what the client might be able to achieve if they can learn to face these experiences in the future. When conducting goal-focused exposure in PCT, the client's most important life goals are explored in depth to help the changes that occur during exposure to be clearly directed to serve the client's real needs.

Within the TCC course, both the Brief Awareness Technique and Goal-focused Exposure are offered to help clients bring awareness to problematic conflicts. Although the brief awareness and exposure techniques are separate sections, they are closely linked because they attempt to reproduce the processes that are active in Method of Levels therapy—sustaining attention on a topic and shifting it to thoughts that are more fundamental to the problem. The Brief Awareness Techniques is designed to help the clients to develop a "window" of awareness that can be brought to bear on the thoughts, feelings, and behaviors involved in conflicted goals. Therefore, the Brief Awareness Technique is delivered prior to the exposure exercise and is shorter than those delivered in some other approaches; for example, MBCT (Segal, Williams, & Teasdale, 2002).

In turn, the Imaginal Goal-focused Exposure then specifically involve encouraging clients to direct attention to experiences and situations in which their most important life goals are blocked. This is likely to involve the kinds of experiences that they normally avoid, but only to the extent that the avoidance blocks important goals (Carey, Kelly, Mansell, & Tai, 2012). For avoidance to be a problem, there will always be an "approach goal" or reason why it is worthwhile for that person to face the avoided experience. For example, someone might avoid presentations for many years, but this would become problematic if they needed to deliver presentations in a new job. Therefore, the focus on goals during exposure enables clients to bring awareness to the most important conflicts. By holding the conflict in mind, this helps the client to establish a new organization of goals that allows them to regain overall control.

We can return to the example of Gemma to illustrate this process. She had a conflict between "I need to express how I feel in relationships" and "I must not upset other people." Ultimately, she realized that both sides were a normal part of feeling worthwhile, and she was then able to be more flexible about meeting these goals and balancing them in different situations. In practice, Gemma managed to generate an image that involved a conflict between her two goals. It was an image of a discussion with a friend in which Gemma had to express some dissatisfaction. She was prompted to remind herself of her goal to be able to feel worthwhile as she held the image in mind. She found that the image changes spontaneously so that she was able to visualize herself being assertive in a way that did not entail upsetting her friend; in fact she found that her friend was empathizing with her. Not everyone will experience such spontaneous changes in their imagery, but the typical process does involve a change in the hear-and-now experience as the exposure proceeds.

This exposure technique is described as "goal focused" in order to emphasize that the function is to promote awareness of higher level goals and the conflict that is preventing these being achieved. This differs from behavioral or cognitive-behavioral approaches, in which the explicit functions of exposure are generally to habituate the client to a feared experience, or to promote reappraisal (Clark, 1986; Foa, Huppert, & Cahill, 2006; Foa & Kozak, 1986; Salkovskis, Clark, Hackmann, Wells, & Gelder, 1999). Both of these outcomes may nevertheless arise from the technique even within this context, but they are not the reason for the technique.

It is important during the exposure exercise that clients feel in control. An experience of being really out of control during this exercise is unlikely to be helpful, as it would perpetuate such feelings and corresponding distress. Also it is likely that the "approach goal," the reason why the client is facing the experience, would be obscured by the short-term experience of extreme distress. For example, the person who is bringing an image to mind of a presentation in front of a huge audience and feels really out of control could find it difficult to maintain their "approach goal" to give a presentation at work. Consequently, the goal-focused exposure technique is framed to encourage clients to choose an experience that provides a personally relevant challenge, but is not so challenging and uncomfortable that they feel really out of control. Also the exposure exercise is self-directed in that prompts are offered, but clients are in control of the experience they bring to mind. In support of this stance most research studies have found that having greater perceived control during exposure exercises reduces anxiety and distress levels (Craske, Bunt, Rapee, & Barlow, 1991; Mcglynn, Rose, & Lazarte, 1994; Rachman, Craske, Tallman, & Solyom, 1986; Rose, McGlynn, & Lazarte, 1995). More recently a study with individuals who feared spiders found that participants with greater control during a computerized exposure task approached closer to a spider afterwards (Healey, Mansell, & Tai, 2017).

## BEFORE THE SESSION

- Set up the room as described in Chapter 4, How to Use This Book, Part A.
- Print out the relevant session handouts (included on the companion website)

- Bring the relevant materials (listed before the condensed session plan on p. 74).
- Put up the continuum.
- Put up the "posters of opposing goals"

## SESSION SECTIONS (OVERVIEW AND STEPS 1–3)

Each major element of the session is described below; wherever relevant we detail linking to previous sections, take home messages, and interactive elements. The "linking between sections" is detailed when it may not be apparent how one section relates to the previous one.

The take home messages are what we broadly want to get across during the section. Individual participants may have their own personally useful take home message. If they express this then this can be useful to explore with curious questioning (see Chapter 4, How to Use This Book, Part A). When clients are filling in worksheets it is useful for facilitators to offer them support as required; for example, let clients know that they can make eye contact with the facilitators or gesture them over if they want to clarify something.

Most session sections have a corresponding PowerPoint slide and section on the worksheet (although this will not always be a section that clients need to fill in). Readers may find it helpful to have the session worksheets in front of them (or periodically refer to them) while reading through the sections. We include examples of worksheets and slides in the main body of the chapter. This is to make clear how these elements fit together, as appreciating this will be vital to smoothly run the Course. Worksheets for this session are on the companion website. The slides for each session are also included on the companion website. Some slides and session sheets are described as "reference" this is used when the slide or sheet is provided for a visual reference but clients do not need to refer to or complete these. The slides are numbered according to the session, step, and slide that they relate to; for example, 1.1.1 would be session 1, step 1, slide 1; 1.2.4 would be session 1, step 2, slide 4. The sheets to give out at the end of the session are described as "additional session sheets" and are also included on the companion website.

### Overview of Session

This introduces the theme of the Course and gives a brief overview of what will be covered during this session. The key theme is control and facilitating people to establish more control over things that are important to them. In doing so, the session also touches upon what blocks control, when attempts at control are problematic and considerations of what would be more helpful on these occasions. As mentioned earlier, it is important not to assume that a particular behavior (or cognitive process) is automatically problematic, but to check this out or encourage clients to check this out. This message can be both normalizing and empowering, giving clients the opportunity to think carefully about how and why they do these things, rather than feeling they must stop doing something that has been part of their way of managing for many years.

Below is an example of the way that this session is introduced. As we mentioned earlier, you do not have to follow what we say to the letter, as you will develop your own style, but having a suggested wording can be useful.

> This course is about how to get back in control of your life. During the course we'll talk about different ways to get more control.
>
> We'll run through eight different steps during this session, looking at different strategies and ways of thinking about things. At the end we'll ask you which bits seemed helpful and less helpful. We can change the things we do next week, so we do more of the things you find helpful. The reason we do this is because we are all different, we will all find different things helpful at different times. It is like we are all experts. We (clinicians) are experts in techniques that can be helpful for people, but you all are experts in your own individual situation and life.
>
> The session will last an hour and a quarter; there won't be a break but if you really need to nip out you can.

## Course Ground Rules

The course ground rules are important to establish early so that people are clear what is expected. We also emphasize clients considering their own level of control within a session so that they feel comfortable. We acknowledge that sometimes it is helpful for people to step outside their "comfort zone," but suggest that this should be done in a way that does not make the individual feel really out of control. The ground rules described below are detailed on a PowerPoint slide, but we also give people the opportunity to suggest other rules if they think there are other important ones.

Below is an example of the sort of thing that you could say—as mentioned previously, these are examples not strict scripts!

> You don't have to share personal experiences, only speak if and when you want to. Anything that a group member says within the session is private and should not be shared with anyone else. Please turn phones off or to silent wherever possible. Encourage you to feel in control of what occurs for you during the sessions, for example, how much you say. You may want/need to slightly step out of your personal comfort zone, but you are in control of whether you do so and by how much.

## Session 1—Step 1: How Much Control Do I Have? A Continuum of Control [See companion website for training video]

### *Materials*

'Step 1—how much control do I have?' reference sheet in worksheets pack
Continuum poster
Pack of large post-it notes
Slide 1.1.3 'how much control do I have'.

This first exercise can involve each person producing his or her own material. People will still be settling into the group, and so it allows for minor to no participation from group members. A PowerPoint slide shows the continuum and this is reproduced on a large piece of paper for the interactive demonstration. Box 5.2 shows a blank continuum at the start of a session.

This section starts simply. The facilitator explains that we all have different degrees of control over different things in our life; this exercise helps to consider how much control we have and which things we can gain more control of. Ideally it is useful if the key "take home messages" emerge from discussions after the exercises. Individual participants may have their own personal take home message.

> *Take home message:* Control is on a continuum or scale. We have different degrees of control over different things. We can all identify things we have little control over, some control over, and a lot of control over. This process of understanding the amount of control we

BOX 5.2

EXAMPLE OF A BLANK CONTINUUM OF CONTROL.

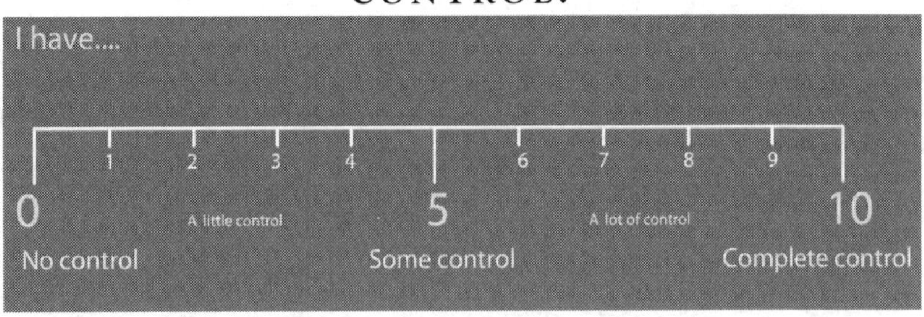

have over different things helps us to manage our lives more effectively.

*Interaction and Feedback:* This section begins with the facilitators reading their own examples. They use post-it notes to denote the amount of control they have over different things in their life. Ideally this would be a "personal" example, e.g., worry, self-criticism, work deadlines. Facilitators can also give a neutral example; e.g., I do not have control over the weather, but can control the impact the weather has on me/how I respond to different conditions, I can wear a coat, check the forecast, etc.

Next, the facilitators ask clients to write down different experiences/situations in their lives and provide a rating on the continuum of how much control they have over this. Again, it is preferable if clients choose examples of things that they want more control over but they can use neutral examples if this makes them more comfortable at this stage. The clients are prompted **not** to include their names. The facilitators ask each client for their permission to put the post-it notes on the continuum that is displayed on the wall. The post-its are put up next to the relevant rating, e.g., if worry is rated as a "3" then the facilitator would stick that post-it next to the number 3 on the continuum. As each post-it note is placed on the continuum at different locations, this should reveal examples of the full range. Facilitators may decide to add more of their own examples to ensure that the full range is illustrated. See Box 5.3 for a completed example of a continuum with a variety of post-it notes of suggestions from facilitators and clients.

*Discussion:* This task is followed by the opportunity for discussion, which may cover a number of areas. Some examples of the types of curious questions that can be used depending on the discussion topics and client utterances that come up are: "Does anyone want to say anything about the rating they chose?" "What are your thoughts on the number you have chosen?" "Is it higher or lower than you expected?" "Does it sit well with you or do you want it high/lower?" "Can you see what higher/lower would look like?"

A common topic of discussion is how clients' ratings compare to one another. Often, several clients include the same experience on their post-it, but give it a different rating. For example, "worry" may be rated as 2, 4, and 5 by different people. These discrepancies provide a valuable opportunity to invite clients to explain their choice of rating. Typically the differences between ratings, and reasons for ratings, prompts clients to reflect on their perceptions of control, which is the aim of the task. For example, worry can be perceived as a choice by some people, but as an uncontrollable habit by others. The facilitators

BOX 5.3

**COMPLETED EXAMPLE OF A CONTINUUM WITH A VARIETY OF POST-IT NOTES OF SUGGESTIONS FROM FACILITATORS AND CLIENTS.**

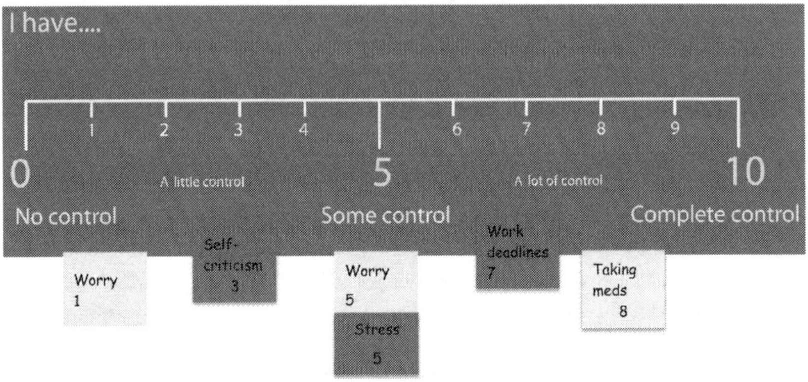


can then explore the reasons with the clients in more detail. It is important to convey that no particular rating is "wrong" or "right." Rather, it is intriguing that the same process can be felt so differently by different people. The facilitators may also mention that the second session explicitly focuses on ways of thinking that can become problematic for people, such as worry and self-criticism.

It can also be helpful for the facilitator to link relevant client comments to the take home message or session themes. For example, it seems to me that what you said relates to our earlier discussion of...? However, it is important to clarify the client's idiosyncratic experience and understanding first by using curious questioning. Otherwise the risk is that the link you suggest will be irrelevant to the client or based on assumption. See Box 5.1 (p. 47) for an example of curious questioning.

Another possible discussion theme can be how clients can respond if they perceive they have no control over an aspect of their life that they would like to change. Again, if someone brings this up it is important to clarify their specific experience and respond appropriately. But a useful suggestion could be to make it explicit that participants can break down goals that seem difficult to achieve, so they can focus on more achievable subgoals. Further, clients may be able to change how they respond to a particular aspect of their life or experience even if they are unable to change the external aspect of their life.

## Session 1—Step 2: Why Do I Want to Take Control of My Problems? [See companion website for training video]

### *Materials*

"Step 2–Why do I want to take control of my problems?" and "What things are most important to me?" worksheets.
"Step 2–Why do I want to take control? What things are most important to me?" Supporting worksheet, with an example and an additional blank worksheet.
Slides (1.2.4 "why I want to take control," *examples*; 1.2.5 "what is important to me"; 1.2.6 "what is important to me, for example").

The purpose of this exercise is to encourage clients to consider what their goals are for attending the sessions and gaining more control of their current problems. This is used as a basis to help people consider their goals more broadly and particularly to explore whether these goals are informed by "deeper" values.

*Take home message:* There are personally important reasons we can all identify for taking control of our problems. It can be helpful to consider what things are really important, as these key goals (or values) drive nearly everything we do. We experience some of our most pressing problems when we are not meeting these important life goals.
*Application and practice:*
We think it is critical to help clients become aware of, and articulate, their main life goals. Therefore, this step includes three consecutive stages that are used to help people elicit them.

1. **Examples and first worksheet section.** The facilitator begins by reading an anonymized list of examples of common reasons that other clients have cited for needing to take control and to manage their problems better. These are shown in slide 1.2.4. It can help to let clients know that the word "problems" is just a term. They might have a more personally meaningful word for what they are experiencing, such as stress, difficulties, or worries. Next, the facilitator asks the clients to fill in their worksheet (Step 2a: "Why do I want to take control of my problems?").
2. **Upward arrow: introduction and complete upward arrow worksheet.** In order to encourage clients to explore their goals in more depth, an "upward arrow" technique is used. Slide 1.2.6, illustrated in Box 5.4, illustrates an example that the facilitators may use at this point. Below is an example of how you could introduce the technique:

> This is an example of one way to clarify the things that are more important to you. We'll try this out in a few minutes and we'll give you a sheet at

## BOX 5.4

### EXAMPLE OF THE UPWARD ARROW ON SESSION SLIDES.

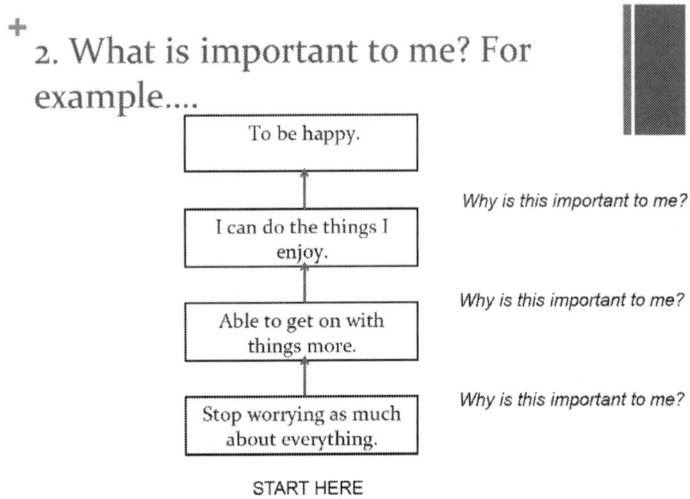


the end in case you want to try this at home. This example is of Kaitlin who wants to stop worrying as much as she is, and what is really important to her about taking control of this. This example is based on what clients who are accessing psychological support have said. [Facilitators talk through the example on slide 1.2.6]:

Kaitlin wrote 'Stop worrying as much about everything' in the bottom box. Then she asked 'Why is 'Stop worrying as much about everything' important to me/ why does this help?, her response was 'I'm able to get on with things more'. She asked 'Why is 'I'm able to get on with things more' important to me/ why does this help? and her response was 'I can do the things I enjoy'. She kept on asking this question until she wrote down a really important basic goal in one of the boxes, 'I want to be happy' and even though she asked 'why is this important to me?' there was no goal more important than this one.

Explain that, similarly, clients will need to identify a goal to include on the worksheet. They will then continue to ask themselves "Why is X *reason/goal* important to me?", or "why does it help?" (the "why is it important question" is usually more useful but occasionally it makes more sense to ask "why it helped"). They keep on asking this question until they write down a really important basic goal in one of the boxes; for example, "I want to be a good parent". These instructions are detailed on the worksheet (see Box 5.5). Facilitators make it clear that clients can make eye contact with the facilitators or gesture them over if they want to clarify something. Occasionally clients will start with a very basic or higher level goal. If this arises the technique can be used to clarify what this means for the client; for example, "what does being a good parent look like?" This involves asking the question "what does that look like, or what does that mean in practice?", instead if "Why is X *reason/goal* important to me?"

Clients fill in the upward arrow worksheet. Please also make sure they have the "Step 2- Why do I want to take control? What things are most important to me?" This is a supporting worksheet, with an example and an additional blank worksheet that clients could use at home if they wanted.

After the clients have completed the upward arrow worksheet, some example questions that can be used to explore client responses' (as appropriate in responding to what individual clients raise) are: "Did you get to the place you were expecting?" "Is where you got to different to where you started?"

3. **Clients fill in third worksheet section.** Having used the upward arrow technique, clients are now asked to complete the second section on their initial worksheet (Step 2b; "What things are important to me? What type of person do I want to be?"); this involves flicking back a page.

   They can use the upward arrow worksheet to inform this. We have found that it can also be helpful to suggest that clients consider the things in their life they value most. For example, the roles that are most important to them, such as being a parent, a friend, or an employee. Offer clients support in completing the worksheets if required; for example, let clients know that they can make eye contact with the facilitators or gesture them over if they want to clarify something.

## Session 1—Step 3: What Causes Us Problems and Blocks Our Control? [See companion website for training video]

### *Materials*

"Step 3—What causes us problems and blocks our control?" reference sheet in worksheets pack.
Elastic bands (fairly big).
Posters that represent opposing goals.

## BOX 5.5

# UPWARD ARROW WORKSHEET.

## Upward Arrow: What things are most important to me?

**Instructions: Upward arrow technique.**

1. Start with the bottom box. Ask yourself:
Why is '*the reason in the bottom box*' important to you/why does this help?
Put your answer in the box above the bottom one.

2. Each new reason that you write, ask yourself the same questions:
Why is '*X*' important to you/why does this help?

3. You can stop moving upwards when you end up with a really important basic goal in one of the boxes, e.g. I want to be happy, I want to be a good parent.

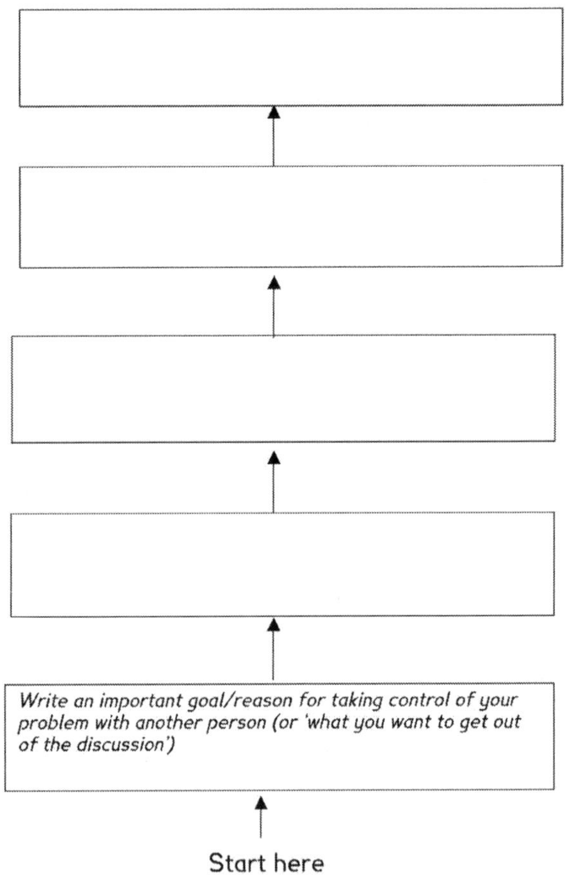

Slides (1.3.7 "what causes us problems and blocks our control"; 1.3.8-10 "what causes us problems," *examples of anger, stress, and sadness*).

This section is about conflict. It introduces the idea that being "stuck between two things" can block control. People may experience being stuck in very different ways. Some people have described it as "knowing what I need to do but not doing it" and as being "pulled around." Being "pulled around" seems to commonly represent the experience of switching between different habits without feeling fully in control or feeling that these habits are helpful. For example, Sonia had an overall higher level goal of "being loved by others." She strived to achieve this socially by going out and drinking heavily with work colleagues. This was only a problem because she also wanted to be highly professional and yet she often found herself becoming overfamiliar in these situations, which led her to worry and ruminate extensively about her conduct. Thus, her ultimate life goal of being loved entailed conflict between the goals of "being intimate" and "being professional." She felt "pulled around" and unable to stay in control. The following exercise demonstrates how conflict can be experienced.

Three clinical examples are prepared and clients can chose which example is focused upon within the below demonstration.

*Interaction and Feedback:*

**1. Introduction (including *Take home message*)**

> Sometimes we experience problems when we are stuck between two different impulses, or two different sides of ourselves. We can feel pushed and pulled, stressed and stretched, but don't always know exactly what is pulling us. We're going to demonstrate how this feeling of being pushed and pulled might play out, in regards to a feeling we might have experienced to some extent. We'd like you to choose whether we focus on anger, stress or sadness, by a show of hands. Please can you put your hand up if you want....

**2. Setting up the demonstration**

Facilitators conduct the elastic band demonstration with the most popular experience. To put the demonstration in context, an example is provided for each experience. Please read out the relevant example (below), depending on what clients have chosen, before completing the elastic band demonstration.

***Anger example:*** *Jo has always tried not to be angry. Trying not to be angry has not been too much of a problem for him, but now he is being bullied at work. He still tries to stop himself feeling and expressing anger, through pushing out his thoughts, criticizing himself, and using alcohol. But he sometimes finds himself intensely angry and believes his* *anger is justified. He both does and doesn't want to feel and express anger and we're going to demo how this can work out.*

***Stress example:*** *Susan has had a number of stressful experiences recently. She doesn't think she should be getting stressed and anxious; she feels she must not worry or let things bother her. However, she also feels she needs to work everything out and manage everything. She moves between distracting herself, drinking alcohol, and trying not to feel any stress and spending hours working things out and feeling stressed.*

***Sadness example:*** *Beth has recently broken up with her boyfriend. She misses him, but feels that she shouldn't miss him, and should just move on. She tries never to cry or feel upset, but finds she sometimes "crashes" and spends hours dwelling on the breakup.*

3. **The demonstration**

The demonstration uses visual representations of the goals (or reference points) described in the above examples. These are on the slides (See Box 5.6), but, for the purpose of the demonstration, facilitators will also need to have them written/printed on paper. See Box 5.7 for a representation of the paper version of Jo's goals, the "anger example." There is also a recording of the demonstration on the accompanying website. Two elastic bands knotted together are used to demonstrate the effect of trying to

BOX 5.6

SLIDE DEPICTING THE EXAMPLE OF JO, THE "ANGER EXAMPLE."

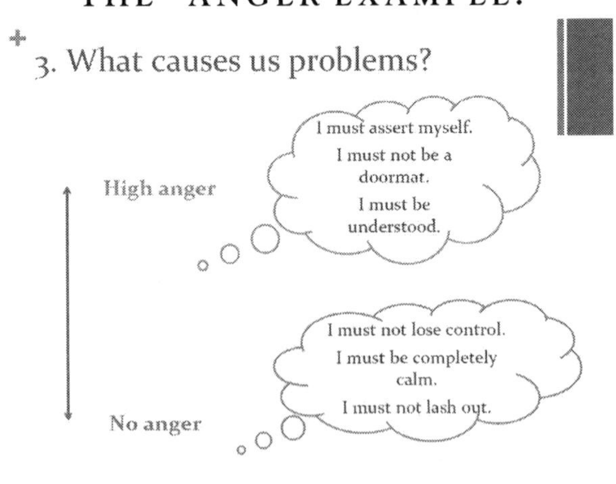

BOX 5.7

**REPRESENTATION OF THE PAPER VERSION OF JO'S GOALS, THE "ANGER EXAMPLE."**

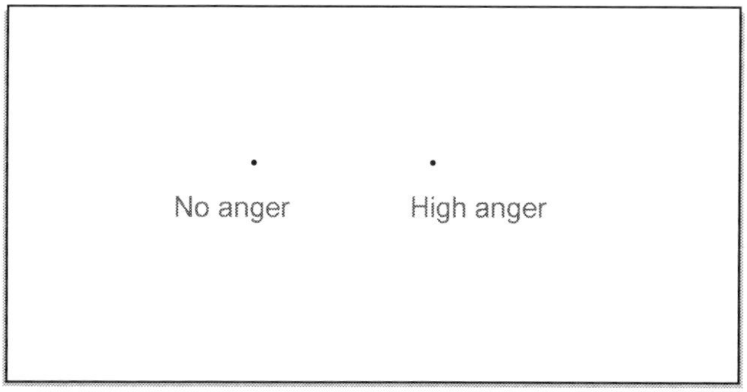


meet both goals at once. The elastic band is used as a visual metaphor for the experience of being pulled in two ways by a goal conflict. But it can also suggest the feeling of being stuck because while the elastic band is pulled in two directions it cannot move in any other direction.

One facilitator will represent one of the goals and the other facilitator will represent the other. The elastic band consists of two elastic bands knotted together and one facilitator will hold a pen in one of the elastic bands and the other facilitator will hold a pen in the other elastic band.

Before doing the demonstration please identify which role you and the other facilitator will play e.g., "I'll represent the goals that lead to 'no anger', Jody will represent the goals that lead to 'high anger'."

To make it clear that the two facilitators represent the conflict within one person, suggest that participants imagine themselves as the knot. Make the link between the thoughts and goals listed on the slides and the relevant feeling; e.g., reading out the goals for no anger, I must be completely calm, I must not lash out, etc. It can also be helpful to read the relevant goals while the two facilitators are conducting the demonstration.

**4. Feedback**

As is appropriate after most of the session sections give participants the opportunity to ask questions or comment. Some example questions that can be used as appropriate are: "How would you describe the band?" "Have you come across this feeling (pushed/pulled)?" "How does it feel to be in between?" "Have you ever felt torn between two things?" "How would it be if the band stayed like this?"

Introduce the idea of checking on their internal elastic band (if this does not emerge from the discussions). The "internal elastic band" can be a useful indicator of how tense, stressed or upset someone is. It can be used to represent the stress that people experience as tension between conflicting goals, or opposing sides of themselves. This can help clients to shift from seeing distressing feelings and experiences as "symptoms" to seeing them as markers of the difficulties resolving important goals they have in their lives. Also it can help explain how the "markers," the distressing feelings and experiences, can change while the problem still remains unresolved. For example, a client could be engaging in rumination regarding feeling under pressure at work—with an underlying conflict "My work must be perfect" and "I must complete all my work fast." After some time of wrestling with rumination they became adept at pushing away their ruminative thoughts using distraction. However, they still felt stressed, flat in mood, and the issue that they were dwelling upon remained unresolved. So, even though the "symptoms" may change, the underlying conflict remains. The symptoms are ultimately relieved when they can bring the original problem to their awareness, and explore the two goals openly.

## HOW TO TAKE CONTROL (STEP 4 ONWARDS)

The remaining sections of this session focus on approaches and techniques that people can use to take greater control over their lives. They focus on raising awareness of their life goals and how the conflict between them undermines their control.

### How to Take Control: Video

#### *Materials*

1.4.11 Video within slides.

The videos depict real people talking about their experiences of various aspects of the problems they were facing or their recovery. They are either people who accessed previous therapy or previous TCCs and have given permission for their accounts to be used in this way. As this is the first video shown, it is worth mentioning that these are real people who have accessed psychological interventions.

*Linking with previous section:* There are ways that we can increase our control over our experiences and move towards our goals. We will be discussing these in the next few exercises in the group.
*Video:* This is a video of Sarah who talks about how she began to get more control over things in her life.

## Session 1—Step 4: How to Take Control: The Three Knights and the Dragon

### *Materials*

"Step 4–How to take control: the dragon story" reference sheet in worksheets pack. Reference slide 1.4.12 "How to take control: dragon." *Facilitators may want to refer to the "additional session sheets" as this details the full metaphor (provided on the companion website).*

As mentioned earlier, the PCT rationale suggests that it is critical for clients to be able to shift and sustain their awareness to their own personal problems for effective change to occur. We have found that a rationale is necessary to justify this to clients in the group. The most accessible way to convey the rationale has been to use a metaphorical story.

The dragon metaphor aims to convey that sometimes it is necessary to "move toward/observe" the things that cause us problems. Avoidance of experiences can cause problems when it conflicts with an important "approach' goal." For example, avoidance of anxiety provoking social experiences can conflict with goals of maintaining relationships, progressing at work, etc. The metaphor draws out the potential goal conflicts that those in the story had. It suggests that flexibility in meeting goals can be helpful when addressing problems. The dragon story also provides a rationale for the subsequent goal-focused exposure exercise.

The story is detailed below; it is informed by a similar story described in Stott, Mansell, Salkovskis, & Lavender (2010):

> Once there was a village at the bottom of a large mountain. There was a fierce dragon lurking in the hills around the village and it has been attacking people. Clearly something has to be done, and so three knights volunteer to help.
>
> Without hesitation, the first knight gets hold of a huge sword and charges in and attacks the dragon. Unfortunately the dragon is too strong for him and frightens him away and he flees the village never to be seen again.
>
> The second knight is really terrified by the first knight's experience and so stays at home. He thinks that he will never be able to defeat the dragon.

The third knight decides he needs more information about the dragon and so he watches the dragon's lair over a number of weeks to find out when the dragon is awake and when the dragon is asleep. He finds out that the dragon goes to sleep at 9pm every night in the corner of his lair. He also asks another knight for help and eventually they are able to sneak up on the dragon and capture it.

*Take home message and linking with previous sections:* We are suggesting that one way achieving what we want, and dealing with any problems that arise, is by approaching and/or observing the things that cause us difficulties.

If we think of the elastic band exercise, the first knight could have had the two goals of being brave and being safe. It seems that the goal of trying to be brave won out against the safety goal! For the second knight the safety goal won out, but the third knight seems to have managed to balance and meet both goals.

Both avoiding problems and going at them full force can be ways we are trying to keep safe. They may not always be the most effective ways of resolving an issue, because it seems that when we have a problem it is helpful to give time and attention.

*Application and practice:* After facilitators have told the story, they can ask clients: "Do you think the third knight and the village were safe after he captured the dragon?"; "Do you think the first two knights were trying to keep safe?" Invite questions or comments, if people want to comment. Then let clients know what the take home messages were if these have not already emerged from the discussion. Some further example curious questions that can be used as appropriate are: "Does anyone have any thoughts on the three knights?" "Can you recognize a time when you have been one of these knights?" "Which knight do you feel had the best approach?" "How do you think the third knight handled the situation?"

Explain that the use of examples and stories is not intended to trivialize problems, but sometimes these can be much easier to remember than a lot of concepts!

## Session 1—Step 5: How to Take Control: The Brief Awareness Technique [See companion website for training video]

### *Materials*

"Step 5–How to take control: The Awareness exercise" reference sheet in worksheets pack

Facilitator "Awareness prompt sheet"

Reference slide 1.5.13 "How to take control: awareness"

The awareness technique is a brief exercise that is focused on attending to sounds. A prompt sheet is provided towards the end of the chapter. If facilitators have not previously led or experienced awareness/mindfulness based practices it is recommended that they listen to examples of these and practice leading the exercise using the prompt sheet. There are a number of examples of mindfulness and awareness practices freely available online; for example, on http://www.freemindfulness.org/download. A metaphor of a train is used to illustrate the "mindful mindset." The theoretical rationale for this, and the subsequent goal-focused exposure technique, were explained in detail towards the beginning of this chapter (p. 48).

*Linking with previous section:* In the previous section we talked about the importance of giving time and attention to the things that cause us problems. This is not always an easy thing to do and in the next section we will practice an exercise that can help us "move towards" or "face" problems or difficult experiences. The awareness exercise develops a "mindful mindset" that can help move towards/face difficult experiences.

*Take home message:* We can make a step toward our important life goals by choosing to face an experience that we have *some* control over right now. This involves facing the experience in a "mindful" way for a period of time where you neither let the experience overwhelm you (losing control completely) nor suppress it completely (try to have complete control over it).

This "mindful mindset" can help you notice what is getting in the way of you taking control. You may notice thoughts, worries or uncomfortable physical experiences are getting in the way of you doing what you want to do. The "mindful mindset" gives you some space to notice the experiences that are getting in the way, without being caught up in the experience or pushing it away.

*Application and practice:* Ask clients to pay attention to sounds in the room, or one particular sound, using the prompt sheet (provided at the end of the chapter). The prompts on the prompt sheet should not be read out like a list, but mentioned with appropriate amounts of space between each prompt.

Please give clients the option of closing their eyes if they want; this can aid concentration but clients need to decide if they feel comfortable with this. Then, after the exercise, ask what they noticed.

Then lead clients through imagining the train, bringing the image to mind (again they can close their eyes). The metaphor models one way of interacting with thoughts/experiences, by noticing and letting thoughts go past.

> Imagine you are waiting on a platform of a small station watching non-stopping goods trains go by.
>
> Each of your thoughts or sensations is like the carriage of a train passing through the station.
>
> There is no point in trying to stop the train or climbing aboard, just be a bystander and watch your thoughts.

Facilitators would then open up for discussion; for example, "How did you find that?" "What did you notice during that?" It is fairly common that clients do not want to talk at length after this exercise and the facilitator certainty does not have to force a discussion if clients are in a "reflective space."

If it does not emerge from the discussion, facilitators can explicitly mention that "paying attention" to an experience is unlikely to be the same as worrying about or dwelling upon a problem. Although such thinking may arise, the instruction is to gently bring attention back to the object of focus. From a PCT perspective, processes that limit awareness of problematic experiences (and related goal conflict) can prevent the process of reorganization and resolution of problems. Both suppression and worry/rumination have the potential to limit awareness (See Session 2). Therefore, in this exercise we are encouraging clients to notice and watch their thoughts and experiences, rather than suppressing these or thinking extensively about them. These ideas are discussed in more detail in the next session, which specifically focuses on thinking that clients are finding problematic.

## STEPS 6 AND 7: GOAL-FOCUSED EXPOSURE TECHNIQUE

There are two sections that apply to the exposure technique. The first helps participants to identify an appropriate experience to use in the second section, which is an imaginal goal-focused exposure exercise. It is important that clients feel in control of the imaginal exposure exercise and do not choose an experience that is so uncomfortable that it will be highly distressing and overwhelming. Therefore, we ask clients to consider the physical sensations associated with the experience as these can influence how distressing an experience is. The theoretical rationale for these sections is explained in detail towards the beginning of this chapter.

## Step 6: Choosing an Experience [See companion website for training video]

### *Materials*

"Step 6–Choosing an experience I want to take control of" worksheet.

Two slides 1.6.14-15 "Choosing an experience I want to take control of."

*Linking with previous* section: A bit like the third knight, in this section we will be getting to understand more about our problems. We will be mapping out the territory and observing a problematic experience. Like the third knight, we may have to observe the problem more than once to help us change it.

*Take home message:* We are suggesting that it can be useful to give our problems time and attention, and to observe problematic experiences. Sometimes we have to observe a problematic experience more than once—this is a step towards resolving the problem. We are going to consider what experience/imagined situation you want to observe as the first step. Generally problematic experiences cause us difficulties because they prevent us from achieving a goal that we value. We will consider which problematic experience/situation is most preventing you from achieving the goals that you value. This can help you decide which experience/situation is the most important one to face as the first step.

*Application and practice:* Slides and worksheets are used to help clients identify the experience/situation that they want to take control of. See Box 5.8 for the slides. Clients are asked to choose an experience that they find somewhat uncomfortable and that is getting in the way of them achieving their valued goals/the things that are important to them. This is an important component and clients can refer back to the goals that they identified in the Step 1 worksheet. It is useful to emphasize that the exercise will be most helpful if clients do not choose an experience that is so uncomfortable that it will be highly distressing and overwhelming.

The slides provide examples of the sorts of experiences clients may want to face, such as feeling of failure, social situations, or a specific recurrent worry. *If facilitators think it will be helpful for their group they can explicitly describe the important goals that these experiences could block (e.g., feeling of failure blocks applying for promotion at work; avoiding social situations blocks building strong relationships; recurrent worry blocks "having peace of mind").*

In order to complete the worksheet (see Box 5.9 for the worksheet), clients consider what physical sensations they might expect when bringing this experience to mind, such as, "heart beats really fast,"

BOX 5.8

SLIDES FOR STEP 6.

## 6. Choosing an experience I want to take control of...

**The Experience**

Think of an 'uncomfortable experience' that is really stopping you from achieving important aims/goals.

Experience: Feeling I've failed at something.

Social situations. Worrying about Jim having an accident.

What kinds of physical sensations might you expect? What kinds of things would you expect to pop into your head during this experience?

Heart beat fast, can't breathe properly. Stomach pain.

Feel really upset and tired.

## 6. Choosing an experience I want to take control of.... (continued)

How long do I think I can face this experience?

Will vary from person to person, depending on the experience.

How comfortable does thinking about this right now make you feel?

0 = "extremely uncomfortable" and 10 = "extremely comfortable".

How comfortable? 0 1 2 3 4 5 6 7 8 9 10

Remind yourself why it might help you to be able to face this experience

I want to be able to enjoy going out. I want to get back to the normal me. I want to feel more relaxed.

"can't breathe properly," "feel really upset and tired." Clients rate the level of comfort for the experience they have chosen and consider if it is manageable. Clients also remind themselves of why they want to face the experience, such as "I want to be able to enjoy going out,"

## BOX 5.9

## "CHOOSING AN EXPERIENCE I WANT TO TAKE CONTROL OF" WORKSHEET.

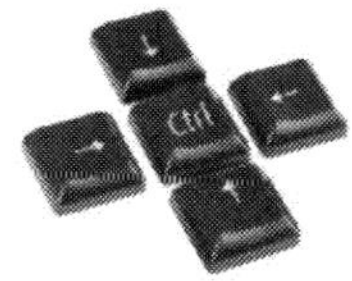

Step 6
Choosing an experience I want to take control of

**The Experience**
Think of an experience that would make you feel uncomfortable, but that you feel you could deal with.
Experience

..........................................................................................................

..........................................................................................................

..........................................................................................................

What kinds of physical sensations might you expect? What kinds of things would you expect to pop into your head during this experience?
Examples include: images, memories, feelings, sounds, impulses and thoughts:

..........................................................................................................

..........................................................................................................

..........................................................................................................

How long do I think I can face this experience?

..........................................................................

How comfortable does thinking about this right now make you feel?
0 = "extremely uncomfortable" and 10 = "extremely comfortable".

How comfortable? 0 1 2 3 4 5 6 7 8 9 10

If the answer is 3 or less you may need to think of a smaller step, or a less uncomfortable, less anxiety-provoking, experience. It can be as simple as looking at a certain object or picture for a certain amount of time.

Remind yourself why it might help you to be able to face this experience

..........................................................................................................

..........................................................................................................

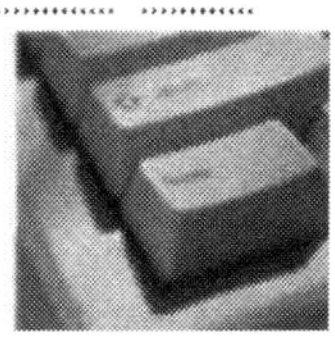

"I want to get back to the normal me." Clients will have considered this earlier in the exercise when they identified the experience/situation that they want to take control of.

## Step 7: Taking Control in Imagination [See companion website for training video]

### *Materials*

"Step 7: Taking control in imagination" reference worksheet.
Reference slide 1.7.16 "Taking control in imagination."
Facilitator prompt sheet: "Guided exposure in imagination."
*Take home message:* Bringing to mind a problematic experience/situation can help us to start to see this differently. Facing these experiences in imagination can also help prepare to face them at other times as this can develop understanding of how in control you might feel and any barriers. By staying with an experience, sometimes we feel a bit different about the experience. This process can enable us to move more fully towards the valued goals that we want to achieve.
*Application and practice:* This exercise involves leading the clients through the imaginal exposure exercise using the relevant prompt sheet (this is provided towards the end of the chapter; p. 77). It is important to make it clear that clients can choose not to do the exercise if the experience they have chosen causes them too much distress. This should be framed by first encouraging clients to try to stay with the previous "manageable" experience that they have chosen, but recognizing that this is the first session and it can be difficult to decide what experience to choose.

Do invite comments or questions about the experience and offer an opportunity for the clients to talk to one of the group facilitators after the sessions as occasionally clients have found this more distressing than they had expected. Example curious questions to use as part of the general discussion, and as relevant to clients, are: "Was this a different way to view what you were thinking about?" "How did you find that?" "What did you notice during that?"

It is useful to again consider the internal process that may occur within this exercise to gain a fuller appreciation of why we frame the exercise as we do. We encourage clients to identify a problematic experience/situation that is getting in the way of them achieving an important goal. Therefore, this will result in clients choosing an experience/situation that they are in conflict about, i.e., one that means they cannot achieve all of their important goals. For example, Roger chose to focus on "anxiety in social situations," as this was blocking his important goal of "Getting a good job." As a first step, he decided to focus on a meeting between six people because this was something he felt a medium level of discomfort regarding. When the TCC facilitator prompted him to consider how he would like the image to be he brought to mind an image of himself "holding the floor" in a confident manner. Although there was no obvious shift in perspective for him this session, in a later TCC session when he repeated this exercise he realized he did come across confidently at this type of meeting. He remembered a couple of recent examples when he had "held the floor" in meetings. After this, he brought to mind more and more challenging social situations during exposure exercises.

## Session 1—Step 8: Summary: Thinking About the Week Ahead

### *Materials*

"Step 8–Thinking about the week ahead" worksheet.
Reference slide 1.7.17 "Thinking about the week ahead."

At the end of each session a brief summary of the session is given. It is also suggested that clients consider what they want to do during the week in order to consolidate the session.

> *Take home message:* It can be helpful to give the things that cause us problems time and attention. This can help us notice whether we are being pulled in two different directions, which can help us feel more in control of what is going on in our lives. Keeping your goals in mind is important because goals keep us motivated to deal with problems. Also we can experience problems when we are not meeting our goals.
>
> During the week you may want to move further towards facing your problems in some way, for example, doing the awareness exercise at home or facing a situation identified for real.
>
> *Application and practice:* Give participants time to look through session worksheets to facilitate them to identify what they want to do at home. We encourage participants to reflect on whether the thing that they have chosen to do will be realistic. We ask them to consider some way of reminding themselves. For example, they might want to set a specific time aside or remind themselves using post-its.

## Give Out Evaluation Form and Additional Sheets

At the end of each session, it is important we give participants the sessional evaluation form and emphasize the importance of feedback. For example, we use the feedback to adapt our style and to shape the content of future sessions. Make the "session 1 additional sheets" available for people to take if they want to (included on companion website).

Provide the overall session themes (in Appendix B) and remind people that they can choose not to attend a session if it does not seem appropriate to the problems that they are working on.

## ALL MATERIALS REQUIRED

**Worksheets required:**

Session 1 worksheet pack
Session 1 additional sheets (to make available at the end of the session)
Session themes (to make available at the end of the session)

**Facilitator prompts required:**

Awareness exercise prompts
Guided exposure in imagination prompts

**Other materials required:**

Continuum control and Post- it notes
Elastic bands (fairly big)
Posters that represent opposing goals
Pens
Projector to show PowerPoint slides and videos
Laptop (to use with projector)
Speakers
PowerPoint presentation
Clinical measures, e.g., measures of depression, anxiety, and functioning (PHQ9, GAD7, WSAS, etc.)

**Optional:**

Facilitator Session 1 guide (in Appendix E)

## DO NOT FORGET!

- Use curious questioning to help clients develop understanding.
- Try to let *take home messages* emerge from client comments/ discussion.
- When responding to the group try to check out what is best for individual group members to enable them to maintain control.
- Be yourself. You, as an individual, will develop your own style of facilitating.

## END OF CHAPTER QUIZ

In order for you to check what you have taken in, we have devised a short quiz. We suggest giving each question a go before checking the answers! (The page on which the answers are located is in brackets after each question).

Describe the concept of control from a PCT perspective? (p. 46; 54; 56)
What is the continuum of control? (p. 54)
What is a goal? (p. 57)
Why is it important to identify goals? (p. 57)
What blocks our control? (p. 61)
What is the elastic band demo? (p. 61–62)
Give an example of a curious question (p. 47; 55)
What is the take home message of the three knights and the dragon story? (p. 66)
Why do we do the awareness exercise? (p. 66)

## CONDENSED SESSION PLAN: SESSION 1

| | |
|---|---|
| Measures | Give participants the clinical measures prior to the session. |
| Overview of Session<br>5 mins | Introduce the theme of the Course and give a brief overview of what will be covered during this session. |
| Course ground rules<br>2 mins | Explain Course Ground Rules: these are on the slides. Give clients the opportunity to add more rules if they think any have been missed. |
| STEP 1. How much control do I have?<br>5–10 mins | Continuum of control exercise. |
| STEP 2. Why do I want to take control of my anxieties/problems?<br>5–10 mins | Includes:<br>– Reasons for taking control on slides<br>– Clients filling in the first section on their worksheet: **Step 2**<br>– Example of "upward arrow" on slides<br>– Clients filling in the second section on their worksheet: **Step 2** |
| STEP 3. What causes us problems and blocks our control?<br>5–10 mins | Includes:<br>– Rationale: experience of being stuck between two things, pushed and pulled<br>– Introduction: demo how feeling pushed and pulled play out. Ask clients to choose focus on anger, stress or sadness |

| | |
|---|---|
| | – Provide relevant example, depending on client choice<br>– Demo: elastic band; both facilitators will be involved in the demo |
| How to take control: video.<br>2 mins | These are videos of real people who have accessed "therapy."<br>Video of Sarah—how she began to get more control over things in her life. |
| | ***SHOULD BE AT LEAST HALFWAY THROUGH*** |
| STEP 4. How to take control: dragon metaphor.<br>5 mins | Dragon story.<br>Qus to prompt discussion: Do you think the third knight and the village were safe after he captured the dragon? Do you think the first two knights were trying to keep safe? |
| STEP 5. How to take control: awareness exercise.<br>5 mins | Includes:<br>– Brief introduction: "mindful mindset"<br>– Awareness exercise<br>– Train metaphor |
| STEP 6. Choosing an experience I want to take control of<br>5–10 mins | Help clients to choose a manageable experience that they sometimes avoid or are having problems with. |
| STEP 7. Taking control in imagination<br>8–10 mins | Use "Guided exposure in imagination prompts" to lead. |
| STEP 8. Summary: Thinking about the week ahead<br>5–10 mins | Brief summary of the session.<br>Clients identify what they want to do at home. |
| Evaluation form and additional sheets | Emphasize the importance of feedback.<br>Provide "session 1 additional sheets" and "overall session themes." |

## AWARENESS EXERCISE PROMPTS

Lead through awareness exercise for 3 minutes. Note: the below are prompts which are not intended to be read out like a list but intended to be "dropped into" the practice at appropriate intervals.

- You may want to close your eyes, you do not have to, the reason I suggest doing so is that it can make it easier to focus on what you have chosen to focus on.
- Become aware of the sensation of contact with the chair
- Try to listen to the sounds inside and outside the room.
- There is no need to listen to particular sounds, you can notice sounds from all directions: sounds that are near or far, in front or behind of you

- If you notice that your mind has wandered bring your attention back to the sounds in the room
- You may also notice the space between the sounds, the silence
- If you notice that you have started to think about other things bring your attention back to the sounds
- In a few moments we will be drawing this practice to a close, so just being aware of this.

## GUIDED EXPOSURE IN IMAGINATION PROMPTS

Lead through awareness exercise for 3 minutes. Note: the below are prompts which are not intended to be read out like a list but intended to be "dropped into" the practice at appropriate intervals.

- As before you may want to close your eyes.
- Can you bring an image of the situation or experience to mind.
- If it is difficult to bring an image to mind, you may be able to get a sense of how you would feel or you could even try bringing a memory to mind.
- How vivid and real does it feel? If it does not feel very vivid you may want to try and imagine sounds or smells, if appropriate, or focus on the colors and details within the image.
- Notice what effect imagining this experience is having on you, on your bodily experiences, on your thoughts. How comfortable do you feel?
- You may need to move the image forward if you have chosen an experience that will change over time and the image is not unfolding naturally.
- If you are able to, you can begin to imagine how you would like the image to be, an ideal experience. Notice what feelings or sensations come with this ideal image or experience.
- Again if this ideal image does not feel real you can imagine colors, sounds, and other details.
- In a few moments we are going to end this practice, so you might want to bring your awareness to the contact of your legs against the chair.

And if you have got your eyes closed, open your eyes.

## References

Carey, T. A., Kelly, R. E., Mansell, W., & Tai, S. J. (2012). What's therapeutic about the therapeutic relationship? A hypothesis for practice informed by Perceptual Control Theory.

*The Cognitive Behaviour Therapist*, *5*(2–3), 47–59. Available from https://doi.org/10.1017/S1754470X12000037.

Clark, D. M. (1986). A cognitive approach to panic. *Behaviour Research and Therapy*, *24*(4), 461–470. Available from https://doi.org/10.1016/0005-7967(86)90011-2.

Craske, M. G., Bunt, R., Rapee, R. M., & Barlow, D. H. (1991). Perceived control and controllability. *Journal of Anxiety Disorders*, *5*(4), 285–292. Available from https://doi.org/10.1016/0887-6185(91)90029-S.

Foa, E. B., Huppert, J. D., & Cahill, S. P. (2006). Emotional processing theory: an update. In B. O. Rothbaum (Ed.), *Pathological Anxiety: Emotional Processing in Etiology and Treatment* (pp. 3–24). New York: Guilford Press.

Foa, E. B., & Kozak, M. J. (1986). Emotional processing of fear: exposure to corrective information. *Psychological Bulletin*, *99*(1), 20. Available from https://doi.org/10.1037/0033-2909.99.1.20.

Healey, A., Mansell, W., & Tai, S. (2017). An experimental test of the role of control in spider fear. *Journal of Anxiety Disorders*, *49*, 12–20.

Mcglynn, F. D., Rose, M. P., & Lazarte, A. (1994). Control and attention during exposure influence arousal and fear among insect phobics. *Behavior Modification*, *18*(4), 371–388. Available from https://doi.org/10.1177/01454455940184001.

Powers, W. T. (1973). *Behavior: The Control of Perception*. Chicago, IL: Aldine.

Rachman, S., Craske, M., Tallman, K., & Solyom, C. (1986). Does escape behavior strengthen agoraphobic avoidance? A replication. *Behavior Therapy*, *17*(4), 366–384. Available from https://doi.org/10.1016/S0005-7894(86)80069-7.

Rose, M. P., McGlynn, F. D., & Lazarte, A. (1995). Control and attention influence snake phobics' arousal and fear during laboratory confrontations with a caged snake. *Journal of Anxiety Disorders*, *9*(4), 293–302. Available from https://doi.org/10.1016/0887-6185(95)00010-L.

Salkovskis, P. M., Clark, D. M., Hackmann, A., Wells, A., & Gelder, M. G. (1999). An experimental investigation of the role of safety-seeking behaviours in the maintenance of panic disorder with agoraphobia. *Behaviour Research and Therapy*, *37*(6), 559–574. Available from https://doi.org/10.1016/S0005-7967(98)00153-3.

Segal, Z. V., Williams, J. M. G., & Teasdale, J. D. (2002). *Mindfulness-Based Cognitive Therapy for Depression: A New Approach to Preventing Relapse*. New York; London: Guilford Press.

Stott, R., Mansell, W., Salkovskis, P., & Lavender, A. (2010). *Oxford Guide to Metaphors in CBT: Building Cognitive Bridges*. Oxford University Press, Oxford.

CHAPTER

# 6

# Session 2 What Blocks Our Control?

## OVERVIEW

In this second session, the focus is on the behaviors and mental processes that can block control. The awareness technique is revisited and it is suggested that this can be used to manage problematic thinking. We also include a range of other techniques.

The format will be the same for all chapters in Part B. The first part of the chapter details the overall theoretical basis of the session and key session sections. Then each session section is detailed, including the materials required for each section. A list of all the materials for the whole session is provided after the session sections. A condensed session plan is provided after the list of all the session materials. Session worksheets are included on the companion website. Slides are numbered by session and order; for example, the first slide in this second session would be 2.1, the second slide 2.2, and so on.

## KEY SESSION FOCUS

A key message here is that thoughts, even negative ones, are not a problem. Even worry, self-criticism, and rumination are normal processes that most people engage in. They are a problem only to the extent that they get in the way of important life goals, or they limit a person's awareness of such goals. This gives clients the opportunity to think carefully about how and why they do these things, rather than feeling they must stop doing something that has been a part of their way of being for many years.

*Transdiagnostic Group Therapy Training and Implementation*
DOI: https://doi.org/10.1016/B978-0-12-813989-9.00006-3

## OVERALL RATIONALE

As we have mentioned, according to Perceptual Control Theory (PCT), conflict is a key cause for loss of control (Mansell, 2005; Powers, 1973). Conflict can occur between people (which we cover in a later session), but the focus of this session is on conflicts that occur *within* a person. The important idea about conflict is that the person holds two incompatible references for how they want their experiences to be. We call these "goals" for ease of use, but people in the group are likely to have different terms for them (e.g., values, ideals, wants, should be's, "just rights", etc.). For example, the experience might be the amount of time spent in the company of other people. A person who says "I need to build up my friendships" and "I want to spend more time on my own" is clearly in conflict over this experience. When goals remain in conflict, it is not possible to simultaneously and consistently pursue both goals. One goal could inhibit the other one; for example, if someone always spent time on their own and did not spend any time pursuing their goal of building friendships. The greater the importance of the inhibited goal to the individual, such as fundamental survival and self-concept goals, the more problematic it will be if the important goal remains inhibited. Many clients we see have deep seated needs to be connected with others, or to feel worthwhile, but their other goals, such as "to avoid rejection," prevent these from being fulfilled.

As detailed in Chapter 2, Conceptual and Theoretical Background and Chapter 5, Session 1 Thinking About Control, reorganization is the process that makes changes to our goals at the point in the control system at which we are currently aware. Therefore it is vital that awareness is brought to the problem. Given that reorganization is a trial-and-error process, it is more likely that reorganization will occur effectively if awareness is sustained. This is because initial changes to goals may not be the most effective. For example, individuals who spend a lot of time on their own may become aware of their conflict between "I need to build up my friendships" vs "I want to spend time on my own," but initial reorganization could lead them to spend all of their time socializing to compensate for their social isolation and then feel so exhausted that they do not enjoy the experience of meeting people, and need to spend even more time on their own. When both goals—to be with others and to spend time alone—are held in awareness and seen by the client as valid parts of the life they want to live, a more balanced resolution is more likely.

It is clear from the perspective of PCT that sustaining present moment awareness on the problem is vital for reorganization to occur and the problem to start to be addressed. This means that any process that gets in the way of awareness going to the problem, and staying there, will slow down successful change, and allow further conflicts to build up unchecked. A PCT account takes the view that the cognitive and behavioral processes that CBT (cognitive behavioral therapy) therapists are familiar with (e.g., worry, rumination, thought suppression, emotion suppression) are problematic when they have such an effect on awareness. They take an individual's awareness away from the source of their problems, and instead their thoughts become focused on noticing their symptoms and how to remove them.

We can see from this perspective that processes such as perfectionism and criticism can be applied in ways that prevent achievement of an important goal. For example, Shafran, Cooper, and Fairburn (2002) have defined problematic clinical perfectionism as "the overdependence of self-evaluation on the determined pursuit of personally demanding, self-imposed standards in at least one highly salient domain, despite adverse consequences" (Shafran et al., 2002, p. 778). This definition emphasizes the continued pursuit of standards *despite adverse consequences*, a "rigid" form of behavior that impinges on other goals (Morris & Mansell, in press). Repeated self-criticism can interfere with the goal of feeling worthwhile, which is a commonly held goal. It is important to note that, according to PCT, such processes will only be problematic for the individual if they block an important goal; for example, perfectionism also has a range of perceived benefits for the individual (Morris & Mansell, in press).

So, it is not the process itself that is "unhelpful" or "maladaptive" in itself. It is relative. Any kind of behavior, mental process, or even personality style is only problematic if they limit a client's awareness of a goal conflict or prevent the achievement of their important goals. Therefore, an important focus of this session is considering what kinds of thinking get in the way of important goals for each individual. Based on this understanding, potential strategies are offered to help manage such problematic thinking, such as awareness exercises and a problem-solving tool with a focus on goal conflict.

The core principle of PCT is that people control their perceptions using their behavior (see Chapter 2: Conceptual and Theoretical Background, Part A). Course facilitators are not exempt from this. We all experience conflict as well as control. Facilitators are encouraged to give "personal" examples during some of the exercises. Personal examples do not mean a detailed account of a very difficult personal problem. For example, there is an exercise during this session (described below) called the PCA problem-solving tool. During this exercise, facilitators are asked to give an example. See Box 6.1 for an illustration of the sort of example a facilitator might give. Providing examples can be normalizing for participants and seems to make the material more

BOX 6.1

**EXAMPLE OF PCA PROBLEM-SOLVING TOOL COMPLETED USING A FACILITATOR EXAMPLE**

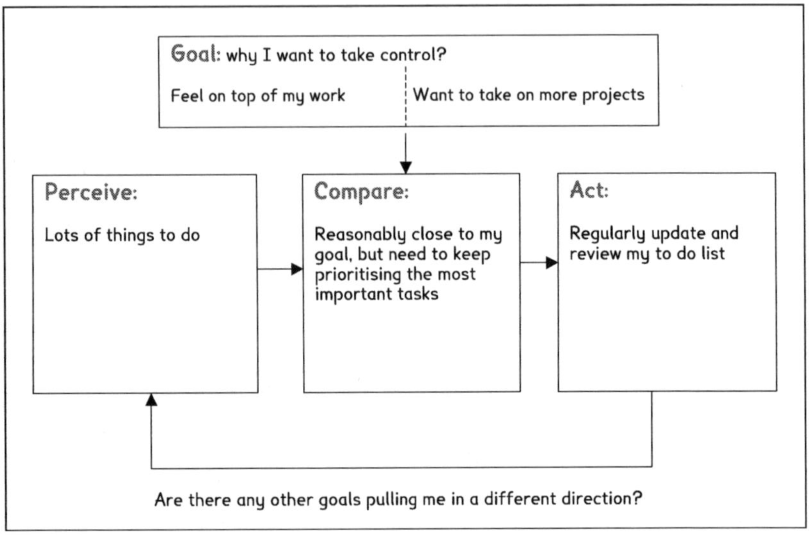


accessible. Participants have consistently provided feedback that they find this useful and have requested more facilitator examples.

## RATIONALE: PCA PROBLEM-SOLVING TOOL

One of the techniques introduced in this session is a problem-solving tool with a focus on goal conflict. You will notice in the problem-solving worksheet that PCA stands for perceive compare act; the origins of these terms are explained in detail in the next paragraph. Although the "perceive" box refers to the problem that is perceived, the word perceive is used to emphasize the normality of the process of control. Even when the effects of the process are problematic it is not that this process is wrong or maladaptive, but that it is not currently achieving the desired effects.

Bill Powers identified three essential aspects for living beings to make events happen the way they want (control). These are perception, comparison, and action (Powers, 1973). Perception refers to perceiving the current experience or situation, comparison refers to the ability to compare the current experience to an internal standard/goal, and then the ability to act enables behavior to make the perception match the internal standard/goal.

Current perception is constantly compared to internal standards, and actions occur to minimize any discrepancies from these standards; in technical terms the discrepancy is described as an error. For example, in a noisy café, a person will speak at a particular volume to make themselves heard, if a noisy group leaves they will reduce their voice so that it does not appear too loud. The reduction in volume occurs because the voice they hear (*perceive*) has become different from their standard for "acceptable volume" (*compare*) and they decrease volume to reduce the discrepancy (*act*). This is described as a *negative feedback loop* because the effect of feeding back is to reduce (or negate) any discrepancy or error. In this example, the negative feedback loop functions to reduce the discrepancy between the individual's current and desired volume. Carey, Mansell, and Tai (2014) review evidence for the role of negative feedback in psychological, social, and biochemical processes.

Although it is not suggested that *negative feedback loops* is a concept that is used while facilitating the take control course (TCC), the idea of perceiving, comparing, and acting is accessible. The PCA problem-solving tool makes explicit a process that happens all the time and applies PCA to a problematic experience or situation. It encourages bringing awareness to a problem and considering the conflicting goals that are present. For example, a client may have a goal of "I want to be trusted by others." The perceived problem is "drinking too much socially causes me to do things I don't feel comfortable with," they compare this to how they want things to be "sometimes I manage not to drink too much but it depends on who I go out with." They could decide on a range of actions, such as "I will leave early when I go out with my heavy-drinking friends" or "I will only take a limited amount of money out so it is less likely I will over-do it." But then, using the PCA tool, they identify that their conflicting goal is "I need to be confident (and drinking helps)." Having identified this, they then consider what actions would bring them closer to both goals.

## BEFORE THE SESSION

- Introducing the problem-solving tool involves giving a personally relevant example. It is really a good idea to prepare personally relevant examples in advance.

- Set up the room as described in Chapter 4, How to use this Book Part A.
- Print out the relevant session handouts (included on the companion website)
- Bring the relevant materials (listed before the condensed session plan on p. 93).

# SESSION SECTIONS

## Overview of the Session

Introduce the theme of the group and give a brief overview of what will be covered during the session. You could say something similar to the below.

"During this session we're going to introduce the idea that individual thoughts, even negative ones, are not a problem; they can be helpful. For example, specific criticism can be helpful- if I'm not paying proper attention when driving and nearly hit someone then I need to criticize my inattentiveness to prevent a future accident. What can be more problematic is repetitive/recurrent and lengthy negative thinking. People end up at places in their heads that they could never get to in reality – far into the future or back into depths of the past. The key issue is that this can block our attempts to do the things that are important to us in the present.

We'll also look at what you can do when you notice a certain type of thinking is preventing you from achieving the things that are important to you."

## What Blocks Our Control?

### *Materials*

Video within slides (2.2 and 2.3).

*Take Home Message:* For many people, there can be certain thinking processes that are problematic. It is useful to consider which thinking processes are problematic for each of us; for example, worry, self-criticism, or dwelling on things. Are these always problematic? Would it still be problematic if we did it less? Can we think of when these things are helpful? It seems important to help each of us to find out what makes these helpful and what makes these unhelpful. This could be different for each of us.

*Application and Practice:* Use the "old women" example to illustrate the difference between "problem-solving" and "dwelling on things" (rumination) (Stott et al., 2010).

"An old women trips on a rug; she can either ask herself why this happened? Why do these things always happen to me? Or she could think: what do I need to do to stop this happening again? How can I rearrange the rug to prevent this happening?"

### *Videos*

The videos are also used to illustrate some of the ways of thinking that can block control.

*Application and Practice:* Show the two video clips: Sarah— "I first started to feel like this"; Sheela—"the mental state I was in at the time." Give clients the opportunity to comment or discuss. Some examples of curious questions that can be used as appropriate are: "Does anything resonate with you from the videos?" "Can you recognize a time you've felt this way?"

## What Blocks Our Control: Self-Criticism

### *Materials*

"Worry, rumination, and critical thinking" worksheet.
Reference slide: "Critical thinking" (2.4).

The cartoon encourages clients to consider how effective self-criticism is. The suggestion being that constant criticism probably will not be too helpful. Although clients may already be aware that constant criticism is not helpful, this exercise encourages them to consider if any criticism is helpful and to consider alternatives.

*Application and Practice:* Use of the cartoon to explore effects of criticism:

"It can be helpful to consider how effective self-criticism will be for you as you are taking control. If you imagine a trial of two different versions of a new teacher training program. In one version of the program they train up the teachers that if pupils are struggling or making mistakes they should be criticized, bullied or called names. In the other version they train teachers to show warmth and encouragement, praising pupils' strengths and supporting them when they are struggling.

Which program produces happier, more confident pupils? If the teachers only gave that children praise and told them what they did was excellent even when they made a mistake, would that be helpful?"

Some examples of curious questions that can be used as appropriate are: "How would you view the two options?" "If it was only positive how would that be?" "Can you see what would be a good balance for you between the two? "Do you think the same approach would be as helpful for other people, as it would for you?"

*Take Home Message:* That constant criticism may not be helpful when experiencing difficulties, trying to learn new ways of managing and taking control. Also that constantly telling ourselves everything we do is excellent may not always be helpful either, as sometimes we need to know/admit when we have made a mistake.

## How to Take Control: Working With Self-Criticism

### *Materials*

"Worry, rumination, and critical thinking" worksheet.
Reference slide: "Critical thinking" (2.4).

This follows on from the previous section; therefore the take home message is similar. In this section, we ask clients to consider which critical things they say to themselves are helpful and which are unhelpful.

*Take Home Message:* That constant criticism is unlikely to be helpful when experiencing difficulties, trying to learn new ways of managing and taking control. But some self-critical thoughts might be helpful so that we know when we have made a mistake and can make changes.
*Application and Practice:* Ask clients to write down the critical things they say to themselves that they feel are helpful and the critical things they say to themselves that they feel are unhelpful. The worksheet also includes some examples of statements that can be helpful in working with self-criticism.

***Optional, judge whether this suits your group*** *(Did they find the imaginal exercise in the previous session helpful? If yes then they might find another imagery-based technique helpful).* The purpose of this exercise is to encourage clients to consider how they can represent problematic thought processes that block control. Ask clients if they can identify an image, or word, or person to represent the critical side of themselves. This could be described as a negative thought monster or self-critical voice. If possible a facilitator example can be used, such as a wicked witch with a very pointy hooked nose and black "lenses" to their eyes. Ask clients to consider what they notice about this image, distinguishing features, and how it makes them feel. There is no worksheet for this, but clients can write things down on the back of other worksheets or facilitators can provide them with blank paper. It is important for the client to consider whether there are any good points of the image. How is it trying to help them, as well as how is it creating problems. We emphasize this in order to encourage clients to maintain a "relationship" with the critical voice/negative thoughts, but one that is more consistent with their own goals. For example, sometimes clients can realize that the wicked witch (self-critical voice) has had a protective function in the past—at times it may have stopped them from making mistakes—but because the witch is a constant critical presence, it undermines their goal of feeling worthwhile.

## How to Take Control: Problem-Solving (PCA) Tool [See companion website for training video]

### *Materials*

"How to take control: Perceive, Compare, Act" worksheet.
Reference slide: "How to take control: Perceive, Compare, Act" (2.5).

This section introduces the PCA problem-solving tool (see Box 6.2 for the example worksheet, clients are also given two blank PCA diagrams as part of the worksheet). This section involves providing a personal facilitator example. We highly recommend that facilitators prepare the personal example in advance; these examples are likely to be much clearer if prepared. The PCA tool is discussed in more detail earlier in the chapter (p. 82–83).

*Take Home Message:* There are some things that we can do something about. But, when there is nothing we can do, it may be more helpful to "let go" or "accept" rather than dwell on these things. Then we can shift attention to a problem that we can start to deal with. You can use the problem-solving approach as an alternative to worry and dwelling. If you realize that there is nothing you can do about the problem then you can use awareness technique and your other resources to help "let go."

When you are struggling with a goal it can be helpful to consider if there are any other goals that are blocking (or conflicting with) this goal. If you think back to the elastic band demo in session 1; when we are struggling with a goal or a problem, there can be conflicting goals causing this.

*Application and Practice:* Talk through how to complete the problem-solving (PCA) tool using a personal example. This is explained and an example is given on p. 83 and a vignette of exactly what the facilitator will say for this example is provided in Box 6.3. It is useful if the facilitator's example considers the effect of the conflicting goal on the actions they have chosen, because awareness of the conflicting goal can alter what the most helpful actions are.

After the facilitator example and explanation of the tool, remind clients that they can consider the problem first (perceive box) and

## BOX 6.2

## "HOW TO TAKE CONTROL: PERCEIVE, COMPARE, ACT" WORKSHEET

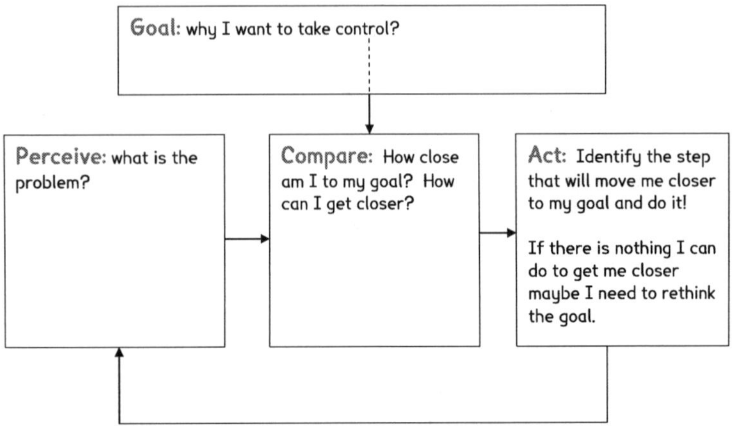


Did what I tried work? Would I do it differently?
Was my goal realistic?
Are there any other goals pulling me in a different direction?

Example:

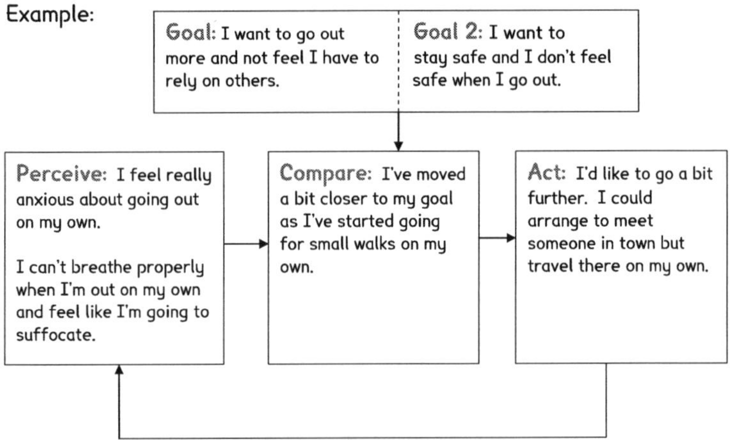


That worked well, I felt better because I knew I was meeting someone.
It meant I could take more risks and it was still realistic.
I also realised that I have another goal to stay safe that was pulling me in the other direction from the goal to go out more (so I added it in as goal 2).

BOX 6.3

## VIGNETTE OF FACILITATOR EXPLAINING PROBLEM-SOLVING (PCA) TOOL

There are some things that we can do something about. But, when there is nothing we can do, it may be more helpful to "let go" or "accept," rather than dwell on these things. Then we can shift attention to a problem that we can start to deal with. We are going to talk through a problem-solving tool. You can use the problem-solving approach as an alternative to worry and dwelling. If by using this tool, you realize that there is nothing you can do about the problem then you can use awareness technique and your other resources to help "let go."

I am going to talk through an example of how I might use the problem-solving tool. I will start by detailing my problem first, but you can start with your goal first if that is easier for you. My problem is that I have a lot of things that I need to do at work and my goal is to feel on top of my work. So I will write the problem in the "perceive box" and the goal in the "goal box." I then want to know how close I am to achieving my goal and conclude that I am reasonably close, but need to keep prioritizing the most important tasks. I write this comparison in the "compare box." Now I think of what I need to do to bring me even closer to my goal and I decide that regularly updating and reviewing my to-do list would be useful and write this in the "act box." If I thought that this wouldn't be realistic because I will forget to do it, I could specify that I will do this on alternate days. Then I check whether there are any other goals pulling me in a different direction and it occurs to me that I have a tendency to want to take on new projects. This makes my to-do list even longer. I can then check how close I am to both goals and whether I need to add any further actions to ensure I meet those. The action I chose before was "regularly update and review my to-do list," but this did not take into account the conflicting goal. Therefore, I can add another action "consider carefully available time before taking on new projects."

then consider the related goal; clients tend to find this easier than considering the goal first. We would also recommend that clients start by filling in only one goal; again this tends to be easier. Give clients the opportunity to fill in the worksheet. Offer clients support in completing the worksheets if required; for example, let clients know that they can make eye contact with the facilitators or gesture them over if they want to clarify something. Once clients have filled in the "goal," "perceive," "compare," "act" boxes, facilitators should prompt them to consider whether there is a competing/conflicting goal; facilitators can use questions, such as "what is getting in the way of you achieving your goal?" and "what is stopping you from doing the things you need to do to manage this problem?" Also prompt clients to consider if and how this conflicting goal would change the actions they have already identified. For example, by saying- "once you have identified the goal that is getting in the way, then it can be useful to consider if you need to change the action(s) you have chosen, so that you can meet both goals."

Following the exercise, the first questions would always be to check understanding of the tool, e.g., "How did you find doing that?," "Did it make sense?," "Did you have any problems filling in any sections?." Other curious questions that can be used as appropriate are: "Were the actions you thought of expected/unexpected?," "Did any solutions come to mind?," "Is there anything in the way of you achieving this other goal (conflicting goal)?," "Did you think of anything additional after recognizing the other goal?."

## How to Take Control: Awareness Exercise

### *Materials*

Facilitator "Awareness prompt sheet"

There are specific reasons for using the awareness exercise in this session, which are described below.

*Linking with Previous Section and Take Home Message:* Sometimes we have problems that we do not have a lot of control over, or that we have done everything we can to solve. But even when there is nothing more that we can do, sometimes we continue thinking the problem through. This can get in the way of us achieving other important goals. By getting better control of our awareness, we can notice when we are doing this and focus on what really matters to us.

*Application and Practice:* Ask clients to pay attention to sounds in the room, or one particular sound, using the prompt sheet (provided toward the end of the chapter on p. 95). Ask what they noticed or whether they have any questions. Then lead participants through imagining a metaphor (e.g., clouds, see below), bringing the image to mind (again they can close their eyes). The metaphor models one way of interacting with thoughts/experiences, by noticing and letting thoughts go past.

Clouds metaphor: Think of your thoughts as clouds floating in the sky. It would be unnecessary and impossible to push clouds away and control their movements. You can imagine your thoughts printed on clouds and allow them to occupy their own space as they pass you by.

## Optional: Taking Control in Imagination

### *Materials*

Reference slide: "Choosing an experience I want to take control of" (2.6)
Facilitator prompt sheet: "Guided exposure in imagination"

Facilitators can decide whether they want to repeat the goal-focused exposure exercise in this session. It is not an essential component, but a PCT approach would suggest it is helpful to keep bringing awareness to problematic experiences until they are resolved. For reorganization and change to occur, PCT suggests that awareness needs to be brought to the "root" of the problem. We gave the example of a client who has a higher level goal conflict between "I need to express how I feel in relationships" and "I must not upset other people." The reader may recall that it was only when she became aware of the "root" conflict that she realized that both sides were a normal part of feeling worthwhile.

*Linking with Previous Session:* You may remember from the first session that we suggested that it is helpful to give the things that cause us problems time and attention. Keeping your goals in mind is important because goals keep us motivated to deal with problems. We experience problems when we are not meeting our goals.
*Take Home Message:* When you bring to mind a problematic experience/situation this can help you to start to see the experience differently.
*Application and Practice:* Remind clients that we did this exercise last week. Use the slide that represents the "choosing an experience I want to deal with" as a visual reminder. Remind clients to think of a problematic experience/situation that is preventing them from achieving important goals. There is a space for clients to fill in the important goal that is being blocked and it is helpful to ask clients to complete this when they write down the "uncomfortable experience." Suggest that they chose an experience/situation that will be manageable and therefore not be too uncomfortable, i.e., around 4/5 level or "medium level" of discomfort. This experience could be something that they currently avoid. It is important to make it clear

that clients can choose not to do the exercise if they realize the experience that they have chosen causes them too much distress.

Lead through the guided exposure exercise using the prompt sheet (this is provided toward the end of the chapter, on p. 95). One way to adapt this exercise for this session theme would be to visualize the critical side of the self/negative thought monster using the examples participants generated earlier in the session. It is best to check with clients what they would prefer. Invite comments or questions about the experience. Offer an opportunity to talk to one of the group facilitators after the sessions as clients could have found this distressing.

## Summary: Thinking About the Week Ahead [See companion website for training video]

### *Materials*

Reference slide: "Choosing an experience I want to take control of" (3.7)
"Thinking about the week ahead" worksheet

At the end of each session, a brief summary is given. It is also suggested that clients consider what they want to do during the week in order to consolidate the session.

*Take Home Message:* During this session, we have considered whether there are ways of thinking, that you as an individual, find problematic. We have suggested that repetitive/recurrent and lengthy negative thinking can be problematic, as people end up at places in their heads that are far away from their current experience and goals. This can block our attempts to do the things that are important to us in the present. Such thinking can also stop us from realizing when we have a conflicting goal that is blocking us from achieving our goals. We used the problem-solving tool as an alternative to repetitive thinking and as a way of checking if we have any blocked goals. We looked at some other ways of preventing problematic thinking from blocking our important goals, such as the mindfulness exercise.

*Application and Practice:* Give participants time to look through session worksheets to help them identify what they want to do at home. We encourage participants to reflect on whether the thing that they have chosen to do will be realistic. We ask them to consider some way of reminding themselves. For example, they might want to set a specific time aside or remind themselves using post-its. Previous clients have put up worksheets that they found helpful somewhere they will regularly see them, such as the fridge door.

## Evaluation Form and Additional Sheets

Give participants the sessional evaluation form. Emphasize the importance of feedback, i.e., we use the feedback to shape the content of the sessions. Make the "Session 2 additional sheets" available for people to take if they want to (included on the companion website).

Provide the overall session themes (in Appendix B) and remind people that they can choose not to attend a session if it does not seem appropriate to the problems that they are working on.

# MATERIALS REQUIRED

**Sheets required:**

- Session 2 worksheets ("Worry, rumination, and critical thinking" worksheet; "How to take control: Perceive, Compare, Act" worksheet; "Choosing an experience I want to take control of" worksheet)
- Session 2 additional sheets ("Worry, rumination, and critical thinking")
- Session themes (to make available at the end of the session)

**Facilitator prompts required:**

- Awareness prompts
- Guided exposure in imagination prompts

**Other materials required:**

- Pens
- Blank paper (in case clients want to note down additional things)
- Projector to show PowerPoint slides and videos
- Laptop (to use with projector)
- Speakers
- PowerPoint presentation
- Clinical measures

# DON'T FORGET

- Use curious questioning to help clients develop understanding.
- Try to let *take home messages* emerge from client comments/discussion.
- When responding to the group, try to check out what is best for individual group members to enable them to maintain control.
- Be yourself. You, as an individual, will develop your own style of facilitating.

## END OF CHAPTER QUIZ

In order for you to check what you have taken in, we have devised a short quiz. We suggest giving each question a go before checking the answers! (Again, the answers are on the page indicated by the number given in brackets).

- Name some processes that can block control. What makes these processes problematic? (p. 81, 84)
- Explain the teacher training program cartoon. What are the take home messages for this section? (p. 84–85)
- Explain the PCA tool step by step and use a personal example (p. 87, 89).

## CONDENSED SESSION PLAN: SESSION 2

| | |
|---|---|
| Measures | Give participants the clinical measures prior to the session. |
| Overview of session<br>*3 min* | Introduce the theme of the session. |
| What blocks our control?<br>*5 min* | Explore characteristics of rumination and worry about the potential impact of these thinking processes. |
| What blocks our control: videos<br>*3 min* | Videos of Sarah and Sheela who describe some of the ways of thinking that blocked their control. |
| What blocks our control: self-criticism.<br>*5 min* | Use the "teacher training program" cartoon to explore effects of criticism. |
| How to take control: working with self-criticism<br>*5 min* | Worksheet: Critical things that are helpful and unhelpful.<br>***Optional:*** Clients identify image, word, or figure to represent the critical side of themselves (negative thought monster or self-critical voice). |
| Problem-solving (PCA) tool<br>*15 min* | Explain PCA problem-solving tool using facilitator example.<br>Clients complete the problem-solving tool.<br>***SHOULD BE AT LEAST HALFWAY THROUGH*** |
| How to take control: awareness exercise.<br>*5–10 min* | Includes:<br>• Brief introduction: using awareness with problematic thinking.<br>• Awareness exercise<br>• Clouds metaphor |

| | |
|---|---|
| ***Optional:*** Taking control in imagination.<br>*5 min* | Facilitate clients to identify a manageable experience.<br>Lead using "Guided exposure in imagination prompts" *(adaptation: visualize the critical side of the self/negative thought monster).* |
| Thinking about the week ahead<br>*5 min* | Brief summary of the session.<br>Clients identify what they want to do at home. |
| Evaluation form and additional sheets | Give participants the sessional evaluation form.<br>Emphasize the importance of feedback.<br>Make the "session 2 additional sheets" available for people to take if they want to. |

## AWARENESS EXERCISE PROMPTS

Lead through awareness exercise for 3 minutes. Note: the below are prompts which are not intended to be read out like a list but intended to be "dropped into" the practice at appropriate intervals.

- You may want to close your eyes, you don't have to, the reason I suggest it is that it will make it easier to focus on what you have chosen to focus on.
- Become aware of the sensation of contact with the chair.
- Try to listen to the sounds inside and outside the room.
- There is no need to listen to particular sounds, you can notice sounds from all directions: sounds that are near or far, in front or behind of you.
- If you notice that your mind has wandered bring your attention back to the sounds in the room.
- You may also notice the space between the sounds and the silence.
- If you notice that you have started to think about other things bring your attention back to the sounds.
- In a few moments, we will be drawing this practice to a close, so just being aware of this.

## GUIDED EXPOSURE IN IMAGINATION PROMPTS

Lead through awareness exercise for 3 min. Note: the below are prompts which are not intended to be read out like a list but intended to be "dropped into" the practice at appropriate intervals.

- As before, you may want to close your eyes:
- Can you bring an image of the situation or experience to mind?
- If it is difficult to bring an image to mind, you may be able to get a sense of how you'd feel or you could even try bringing a memory to mind.

- How vivid and real does it feel? If it doesn't feel very vivid you may want to try and imagine sounds or smells if appropriate, or focus on the colors and details within the image.
- Notice what effect imagining this experience is having on you, on your bodily experiences, on your thoughts. How comfortable do you feel?
- You may need to move the image forward if you have chosen an experience that will change over time and the image is not unfolding naturally.
- If you can begin to imagine how you'd like the image to be, an ideal experience. Notice what feelings or sensations come with this ideal image or experience.
- Again if this ideal image doesn't feel real you can imagine colors, sounds, and other details.
- In a few moments, we are going to end this practice, so you might want to bring your awareness to the contact of your legs against the chair.

And if you've got your eyes closed, open your eyes.

## References

Carey, T. A., Mansell, W., & Tai, S. J. (2014). A biopsychosocial model based on negative feedback and control. *Frontiers in Human Neuroscience, 8*, 94. Available from https://doi.org/10.3389/fnhum.2014.00094.

Mansell, W. (2005). Control theory and psychopathology: An integrative approach. *Psychology and Psychotherapy-Theory Research and Practice, 78*, 141–178. Available from https://doi.org/10.1348/147608304x21400.

Morris, L., & Mansell, W. (in press). A systematic review of the relationship between rigidity/flexibility and transdiagnostic cognitive and behavioral processes that maintain psychopathology. Psychopathology Review.

Powers, W. T. (1973). *Behavior: The control of perception*. Chicago, IL: Aldine.

Shafran, R., Cooper, Z., & Fairburn, C. G. (2002). Clinical perfectionism: A cognitive-behavioural analysis. *Behaviour Research and Therapy, 40*(7), 773–791. Available from https://doi.org/10.1016/S0005-7967(01)00059-6.

CHAPTER

# 7

# Session 3 Feeling in Control Short Term vs Getting Control of Your Life

## OVERVIEW

This third session focuses upon considering the relative importance of short- and long-term goals. It enables clients to weigh up which goals are most important to them and consider prioritizing the most important.

The format will be the same for all the chapters in Part B. The first part of the chapter details the overall theoretical basis of the session and key session sections. Then each session section is detailed, including the materials required for each section. A list of all the materials for the session is provided after the session sections. Slides are numbered by session and order; for example, the first slide in the third session would be 3.1, the second slide 3.2. A condensed session plan is provided after the list of all the session materials. Session worksheets are included on the companion website. When clients are filling in worksheets, it is useful for facilitators to offer them support as required; for example, let clients know that they can make eye contact with the facilitators or gesture them over if they want to clarify something.

## KEY SESSION FOCUS

A fundamental message of the session is that sometimes our attempts to control our emotions, avoid distress, or keep safe can actually get in our way of doing things that are helping us keep in control of our lives as a whole. This session gives clients the opportunity to consider if there

*Transdiagnostic Group Therapy Training and Implementation*
DOI: https://doi.org/10.1016/B978-0-12-813989-9.00007-5

are any important long-term (or higher level) goals that are being blocked by short-term ones that are relatively less important. This encourages clients to focus on their longer term goals and to consider how to prioritize these over short-term goals that are getting in the way.

## OVERALL RATIONALE: HIERARCHIES REVISITED

The principle of a hierarchy provides a key basis of this session. The readers may recall that perceptual control theory (PCT) suggests that our goals are organized hierarchically; this means that goals are represented at different levels. Higher level, long-term goals lead to the setting of subgoals that in turn regulate lower level, shorter term goals. For example, a higher level goal of "being a successful person" could lead to the setting of subgoals, such as "meeting work deadlines," and this in turn could lead to the setting of lower level goals, such as "stay late to work on an important project." Therefore, for any goal or problem that is being discussed, there are likely to be successively higher levels that indicate why this is important, and lower levels that describe how to implement actions to achieve the goal. Experiences are monitored against the higher level goal in order to ascertain whether this goal is being achieved.

Conflicts within the hierarchy cause psychological distress and symptoms. From a PCT perspective, conflict involves three or more layers of the control hierarchy (Mansell, 2012). Signals from the upper level are sent to the next level down, and these can result in incompatible goals being set. For example, someone may try to be a good person (upper level goal) by helping their friends and spending time with their family (mid-level goals). These goals could conflict if a friend became particularly reliant on them, leaving them less time to spend with their family. This "mid-level" would then send signals to the level below and the fact that incompatible goals were being specified would mean that the signal would vary unpredictably. Therefore, they might feel quite torn and vacillate between spending time talking to their friend and not picking up their calls. The conflict would only be resolved when the highest level alters its signal, i.e., when there is change (reorganization) at the highest level that is setting the conflict in motion.

Within the session, a distinction is introduced between short- and long-term goals. Long-term goals represent higher level goals; for example, "I want to have a good relationship with my family," "I want to be a good friend," and "it is important for me to do well at work." Such higher level goals can sometimes be described as values or principles and include self-concept goals; for example, "it is important that I'm a good parent," and "I want to be a successful person." This distinction is used to encourage clients to consider whether they are meeting their higher level or longer term goals and where there are any short-term goals that are getting in the way. For example, a common short-term goal that can prevent achievement of long-term goals is "I must avoid all distress/anxiety." Clients experiencing social anxiety/phobia symptoms often avoid social situations in order to try to avoid experiencing the anxiety evoked by these situations. A more specific example is a client called Abdel who avoided thinking about or experiencing any situations at work that he found difficult. He struggled particularly with interactions with senior colleagues and would cancel appraisal meetings or other interactions. In the short term, he felt OK because he did not have to experience any of the worry, feelings of failure, and anxiety that accompanied these situations. However, in the long term, he was not able to progress within his career, as he was not able to discuss his performance and senior colleagues perceived him to be unreliable.

Ultimately, it is the higher level conflicts that are setting the shorter term goals that would need to be resolved. Returning to the example of Abdel, it was not until he became aware of a conflict between goals of "I must never admit that my performance isn't perfect" and "I need to share how I'm doing to obtain support" that he was able to change his perspective. By reflecting on the anxiety and worry that he was experiencing short term, he not only realized that these resulted from fear that senior colleagues would see that his work was not perfect, but he also realized that actually nobody in the company was perfect. Therefore, he was able to discuss his performance more openly. So even in this session, the distinction between short- and long-term goals is used as a medium to enable clients to reflect on what goals are getting in the way of their higher level goals and to bring awareness to higher level conflicts.

Again it is important to note that from a PCT perspective, it is not that avoidance of certain situations and emotions is always problematic, but this becomes problematic when it blocks important goals. For example, it could be adaptive to avoid a particular individual at work who has a very negative and aggressive attitude. However, this could become problematic if the individual avoided any possible social opportunities at work in case the aggressive colleague was present. This would undermine the goal of "maintaining good relationships with colleagues." So a key theme of this session is encouraging clients to evaluate how beneficial certain actions and responses are and whether these enable the achievement of important goals or stand in the way of them.

## RATIONALE: UNDERSTANDING EMOTIONS

A number of accounts, including PCT, suggest that "negative" emotions arise in response to perceiving stimuli in order to prepare the individual for action and meeting a goal (Frijda, 1986; Gross & Thompson, 2007; Magen & Gross, 2010; Powers, 2005). The term negative is used here to distinguish emotions (e.g., anger, fear, and depression) from emotions, which are often described as pleasant, that do not promote the same tendency toward action (e.g., contentment, equanimity) (Powers, 2008). In addition to specifying that such "negative" emotions prepare for meeting a goal, a PCT account specifies that these arise when there is error within the system (Powers, 2005). Error refers to the signal within the individual that something is "not right" or discrepant (error was also described in Chapter 2, Part A and Chapter 6, Part B). Error signals that there is a conflict and is experienced as a loss of control. For example, irritation at being stuck in a traffic jam signals that my goal of "getting to where I want to go" is not being met. The irritation arises because there is error or, to put it another way, the current situation is discrepant with my goal. Eventually, the traffic will subside and therefore this irritation, as an immediate response to the error, would be short lived. Negative emotions are seen as functional markers that a goal is not being achieved and can dissipate on their own when this is achieved.

Emotions endure when the goal is not (or cannot be) pursued and the error cannot be corrected (Powers, 2005), i.e., at times of loss of control. For example, despondency/depression may arise in response to a poor job interview performance and could persist if the individual does not attend any further interviews (unless they no longer want to get a new job). Even in this scenario, it is not that the emotion is abnormal; it is still serving the function of alerting the individual to error. But they may need some support to identify how to reduce this error. When "negative" emotions endure, this can be a powerful indicator that an important goal is not being met. However, there are some ways in which we can try to manage our emotions that ignore the underlying function of these. For example, Jane started taking beta-blockers to manage anxiety. One of the times that she felt particularly anxious was when she was driving; so she started taking beta-blockers before drives. However, she found that she needed some anxiety to drive well because when another car pulled in front of her (or a similar threat arose), she needed the instinctive anxiety response to quickly react. Without this, she found she was responding much more slowly to threats when driving and risked causing an accident. Part of the theme of this session is encouraging participants to reflect whether any of their strategies/responses could be preventing them from achieving their long-term goals. Again it is not that we are suggesting that emotional suppression is always unhelpful but rather encouraging each individual to establish the function (or lack of function) for them. This could be situation and context dependent; for example, following a bereavement, one might suppress some of the feelings of grief while at work but express these to close friends and family.

## BEFORE THE SESSION

- Introducing the "Short-term, long-term worksheet" involves giving a personally relevant example. It is good to prepare personally relevant examples in advance.
- Set up the room as described in Chapter 4, How to Use This Book, Part A.
- Print out the relevant session handouts (listed before the condensed session plan on p. 107).
- Bring the relevant materials (listed before the condensed session plan on p. 107–108).

## SESSION SECTIONS

### Overview of Session

Introduce the theme of the group and give a brief overview of what will be covered during the session. You could say something similar to the following:

Sometimes (not always) our attempts to control our emotions, avoid distress, or keep safe can actually get in our way of doing things that give us better control over our lives in the long term. For example, avoiding social situations, because these make us feel anxious, will get in the way of meeting new people. Sometimes, it seems like we have to let go of control a little in the short term and experience some discomfort for long-term benefit.

### What Do We Often Try to Control? The Fight-or-Flight Response

***Materials:***

"What do we often try to control? The fight-or-flight response" worksheet.

Reference slide: "What do we often try to control? The fight-or-flight response" (3.2).

*Application and practice:* Give clients more information about the fight-or-flight response, saying something similar to the below:

> When we encounter a potential threat to our survival, our body prepares to counteract this with the 'fight-or-flight' response. In order to help us prepare to run or fight in response to threats, our bodies react by secreting hormones, which quickly begin to have noticeable effects.

The heart starts to beat more quickly and we start to breath more quickly; this is to enable more blood and oxygen to be pumped to the muscles. Muscles tense and can produce stabbing pains. These experiences, or other experiences trigged by the flight or fight response, can feel frightening but they are a normal response to threat.

Give out the fight-or-flight worksheet and ask participants to fill in the experiences that they notice when they're anxious (or angry).

*Linking with theme and take home message:* The fight-or-flight response is a natural physical — way that the body prepares to deal with a threat so it often arises when we feel anxious or angry. But it can feel quite uncomfortable. Sometimes we try to control the physical effects of the fight-or-flight response, perhaps in order to stop the sensations that make us feel uncomfortable. However, these attempts to control can actually prolong our physical response! In this example, we need to experience the physical anxiety short term so that we can feel less anxious longer term. Some curious questions that can be asked of the group, as relevant to their communications and queries, are as follows: "Have you ever experienced these sensations?" "Can you think of a time you've experienced this?" "Do you think it could be this response?"

## Designing a Human Being from Scratch

***Materials:***

Outline of the upper body of a full-size person (e.g., either drawn onto a large piece of paper or whiteboard)

Post-its

*Application and practice:* Ask the group, if they were to design a balanced human being from scratch, what emotions (both positive and negative) would they give the person and why. Facilitators give examples, one "positive" and one "negative" and write on post-its. It is useful if facilitators give a short explanation of why they are "giving" the human being that emotion; for example, "anger because you sometimes need to be able to stick up for yourself." Then ask clients to write one or two examples on post-its. After sticking all the post-its onto the outline of the body, ask clients whether anyone wants to say why they have "given" the human being the emotion they have chosen.

*Linking with theme and take home message:* This brings out from people the normality, and more importantly the functionality, of emotions. Often clients will observe that some of the emotions that they do not want to experience can be helpful. Again this can be an opportunity to use some curious questioning to explore individuals' responses to certain emotions.

There are a couple of ways to explicitly link this with "short-term, long-term" theme. One is that in the short term, our emotional experiences may seem uncomfortable or unpleasant but are useful overall and longer term. Sometimes a theme emerges that emotional suppression can be quite effective short term but can be unhelpful as a longer term approach to emotions. This relates to the point that emotions are normal, and sometimes by letting them run their course, they naturally subside over time, e.g., the fight-or-flight response naturally subsides once the threat is gone. However, another theme that can emerge is clients describing difficulties with particular "negative" emotions, which are difficult because the emotions are enduring. The most useful approach is likely to be asking the individual about this difficulty in a curious way. From a PCT perspective, we would predict that the fact that the "negative" emotion endured indicates that the individual was not meeting all of their important goals.

Some examples of curious questions that can be used as appropriate are as follows: "What are your thoughts on the overall spread of these post-its?" "Does it seem balanced?" "How would balance be for you?" "Anything extra needed to be more balanced?" "Do you feel all these emotions are needed?" "Are 'negative emotions' always negative?" "Are any negative emotions useful?"

## Video

***Materials:***

Video of Sarah, slide "short term vs long term: Sarah" (3.3)

The video includes Sarah talking about trying to hide the fact she was feeling really anxious.

After the video, you can ask clients some "prompt questions." Do you think hiding anxiety was helpful for Sarah in long term? Do you think it was helpful for her in short term? Sometimes clients may want to discuss other areas that relate to Sarah's experience; for example, she talks about feeling like a different person, like there was something wrong, but felt uncomfortable sharing this with other people.

## Short Term vs Long Term [See companion website for training video]

***Materials:***

Short- vs long-term worksheet
Reference slides: "Short term vs long term" (3.4–3.5)

*Link to previous sessions and take home message:* In previous sessions, we have talked about the importance of our goals. Our goals tend to keep us motivated to face challenges. In this section, we are going to consider if there are any things that we do in the short term that get in the way of us achieving the goals that are really important to us.

Sometimes we might choose to prioritize our long-term goals even if this causes us some short-term distress or anxiety. We are going to read an everyday example that illustrates this, but we are aware that you are unlikely to be struggling with this kind of distress!

I don't find cutting onions pleasant at all and often end up with crying eyes. However, if I'm preparing a special dinner for friends, it's more important to me to ensure that my friends have a great meal than removing the irritation of briefly stinging eyes by not cutting up the onions.

*Application and practice:* Demonstrate completing the "short- vs long-term" worksheet using a personal example. (Note: It is really important to clearly decide on the example as this is a relatively complex worksheet and facilitators have to be able to explain it clearly.) A facilitator example is provided in Box 7.1 on the "short- vs long-term" worksheet.

BOX 7.1

## SHORT- VS LONG-TERM WORKSHEET WITH FACILITATOR EXAMPLE

**Short term vs long term**

Why do I want to take control of my anxieties/ problems?

Keep my friendships

| What I do now? | Short term | | Long term | |
|---|---|---|---|---|
| | Pros | Cons | Pros | Cons |
| Arrive late so not waiting on my own | Don't feel uncomfortable | Annoys some of my friends | | Has a negative impact on some friendships |
| Cancel meeting people if tired or don't feel up to it | Can have a rest and don't have to go out when tired | Annoys friends. They can feel let down | | Risk loosing some friendships |

Is there anything I want to do differently......?

I think I should be more careful when I arrange things that I can definitely commit, so I don't have to cancel last minute.

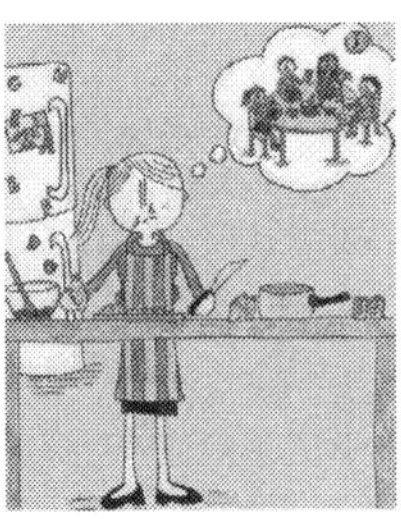

'Letting go' in the short run to make it in the long run

"I don't find cutting onions pleasant at all and often end up with crying eyes. However, if I'm preparing a special dinner for friends it's more important to me to ensure that my friends have a great meal than removing the irritation of briefly stinging eyes by not cutting up the onions."

Ask clients to complete "Short- vs long-term worksheet." The first step is to identify a really important reason why they want to take control of their anxieties/problems, e.g., want to be happy. *Facilitators can refer to the upward arrow technique introduced in the first session.* Then clients identify whether their strategies, responses, or current ways of managing have short- (e.g., make them feel better) or long-term benefits (e.g., move them toward their goals). Finally, clients consider whether there is anything that they could do differently that would help them toward their most important goals.

Some curious questions that can be used as appropriate are the following: "Do you recognize any short-term actions that are having long-term consequences?" "Do any short-term actions have long-term gains?" "Do any short-term actions impact on your overall goals?" "Do you need to change or adapt any short-term actions?" "Does changing or adapting some short-term actions have a positive impact?" "Does adapting/changing produce any long-term gains?"

## How to Take Control: Awareness Exercise

***Materials:***

Body awareness prompts

In this session, the awareness practice is body based (see prompt sheet toward the end of the chapter, p. 109–110). A body-based awareness practice is introduced in this session as the fight-or-flight response was explained earlier. So if clients become aware of any uncomfortable bodily anxiety symptoms, they will be able to understand these as the fight-or-flight response.

*Take home message and link to previous sections:* Awareness techniques can help us notice our emotions and experiences without feeling that we have to change them. Having a "mindful mindset" can help us to experience short-term discomfort in order to meet longer term goals, without being overwhelmed or pushing away those experiences.
*Application and practice:* Ask participants to pay attention to sensations in body (they can close their eyes if they want), then ask what they noticed. It can be worth mentioning that the intention of the practice is not to feel relaxed or calm, although this may happen, the intention of the practice is to bring awareness to the sensations you notice. Lead participants through imagining a metaphor, bringing the image to mind as part of the awareness practice (see Appendix F for examples of metaphors). The metaphor models one way of interacting with thoughts and experiences, by noticing and letting thoughts go past.

## Taking Control in Imagination

***Materials:***

Reference slide: "Choosing an experience I want to take control of" (3.6)
"Choosing an experience I want to take control of" worksheet
Facilitator prompt sheet: "Guided exposure in imagination"
*Take home message and link to previous sections:* It can be difficult to experience short-term discomfort, even it helps us to achieve something that is really important to us. By using the "mindful mindset," we can observe an uncomfortable experience in imagination, and this can help us observe such experiences at other times.
*Application and practice:* Use the slide "Choosing an experience I want to take control of" (see Box 7.2) to encourage clients to think of an uncomfortable experience that is preventing them from achieving important goals. There is a space for clients to fill in the important goal that is being blocked, and it is helpful to ask clients to complete this when they write down the "uncomfortable experience." The experience chosen should be an experience/situation that is around a

BOX 7.2

EXAMPLE OF "CHOOSING AN EXPERIENCE I WANT TO TAKE CONTROL OF" SLIDE

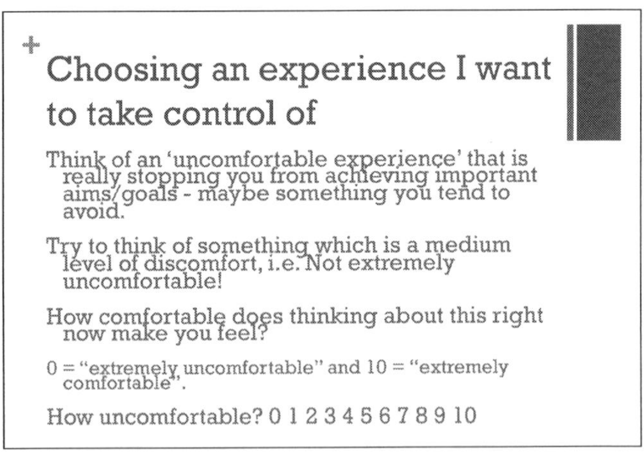

4/5 level of discomfort, or "medium level" of discomfort. The important thing is that the experience is not so challenging and uncomfortable that it will be overwhelming.
Lead through the guided exposure exercise using the prompt sheet (this is provided toward the end of the chapter). Invite comments or questions about the experience. Offer an opportunity to talk to one of the group facilitators after the sessions as clients could have found this distressing.

## Thinking About the Week Ahead

***Materials:***

Reference slide: "Thinking about the week ahead" (3.7)
"Thinking about the week ahead" worksheet

At the end of each session, a brief summary is given. It is also suggested that clients consider what they want to do during the week in order to consolidate the session.

*Take home message:* We noticed that in the short term, some of our feelings can seem uncomfortable or unpleasant but can be useful overall and longer term. We practiced ways of clarifying whether the things we do move us toward our goals or if they only benefit us short term. Sometimes it seems like we have to let go of control a little in the short term and experience some discomfort for long-term benefit.
*Application and practice:* Encourage participants to fill in the "Thinking about the week ahead" worksheet. Encourage them to include specific goals and ways of remembering these as appropriate. For example, they might want to take an initial realistic step toward a long-term goal that they have recognized is important.

# MATERIALS REQUIRED

**Worksheets required:**

"What do we often try to control? The fight-or-flight response" worksheet.
"Short- vs long-term" worksheet
"Choosing an experience I want to take control of" worksheet.
"Thinking about the week ahead" worksheet
Session 3 additional sheet: "What do we often try to control? The fight-or-flight response"

**Facilitator prompts required:**

Body awareness prompts
Guided exposure in imagination prompts

**Other materials required:**

Post-its
Body online drawn on paper, or whiteboard pens to draw on whiteboard (if available)
Pens
Projector to show PowerPoint slides and videos
Laptop (to use with projector)
Speakers
PowerPoint presentation
Clinical measures

## DON'T FORGET

- Use curious questioning to help clients develop understanding.
- Try to let *take home messages* emerge from client comments/ discussion.
- When responding to the group, try to check out what is best for individual group members to enable them to maintain control.
- Where appropriate, link each session to previous sessions or session sections.

## END OF CHAPTER QUIZ

In order for you to check what you have taken in, we have devised a short quiz. We suggest giving each question a go before checking the answers!

Explain the rationale for examining short- and long-term goals (p. 98–99)
Explain the fight/flight response (p. 101)
Why do we "design a human body from scratch?" (p. 102–103)
Explain the rationale for taking control in imagination? (p. 106)

## CONDENSED SESSION PLAN: SESSION 3

| | |
|---|---|
| Measures | Give clients the clinical measures prior to the session |
| Theme<br>*3 min* | Introduce the theme of the session |
| Fight-or-flight response<br>*5–10 min* | Includes the following:<br>• Providing information about fight-or-flight response<br>• Fight-or-flight worksheet |
| Designing a human being from scratch<br>*5–10 min* | Designing a balanced human being: what emotions (both positive and negative) would the group give the person and why<br>• Provide facilitator examples of emotions<br>• Ask clients to write examples on post-its |
| Video<br>*3–5 min* | Sarah talking about trying to hide the fact she was feeling really anxious<br>• Show video and then ask prompt questions |
| Short- vs long-term worksheet<br>*5 min* | Provide facilitator example of "short- vs long-term worksheet" and then ask clients to complete worksheet<br>***SHOULD BE AT LEAST HALFWAY THROUGH*** |
| How to take control: awareness exercise<br>*5–10 min* | Includes the following:<br>• Brief introduction: using awareness with distressing experiences<br>• Body awareness exercise |
| Taking control in imagination<br>*5 min* | Facilitate clients to identify a manageable experience<br>Lead through exercise using "Guided exposure in imagination prompts" |
| Thinking about the week ahead<br>*5 min* | Brief summary of the session<br>Clients identify what they want to do at home |
| Evaluation form | Give participants the sessional evaluation form |

## BODY AWARENESS

Lead through awareness exercise for 3 min. Note: The following are prompts that are not intended to be read out like a list but intended to be "dropped into" the practice at appropriate intervals.

You may want to close your eyes—you don't have to—the reason I suggest it is that it can make it easier to focus on what you have chosen to focus on.

- Take a few moments to become aware of the movement of your breath and the physical sensations in the body.
- When you are ready, bring your awareness to the sensations of touch and pressure where your body makes contact with the chair.
- Now bring your awareness to your feet, feel any sensations in the feet.
- It is likely that your mind will wander from time to time, and if it does, just notice it and gently return your attention to the part of the body you are focusing on.
- Bringing awareness to your lower leg, the calf, shin, and knee. You might notice sensations of your clothes against your skin or you might notice other sensations.
- If you become aware of any tension in the body, you can breathe into them, using the in-breath to gently bring awareness into the sensations.
- Allowing your awareness to move up the body, to the abdomen or stomach area. Become aware of the changing pattern of sensations in the abdominal wall as you breathe in and breathe out.
- In a few moments, we'll be drawing this practice to a close, so just being aware of this.
- When you are ready, open your eyes and bring your attention back to the room.

## GUIDED EXPOSURE IN IMAGINATION PROMPTS

Lead through awareness exercise for 3 min. Note: The following are prompts that are not intended to be read out like a list but intended to be "dropped into" the practice at appropriate intervals.

As before, you may want to close your eyes.

- Can you bring an image of the situation or experience to mind?
- If it is difficult to bring an image to mind, you may be able to get a sense of how you'd feel or you could even try bringing a memory to mind.
- How vivid and real does it feel? If it doesn't feel very vivid, you may want to try and imagine sounds or smells if appropriate or focus on the colors and details within the image.
- Notice what effect imagining this experience is having on you, on your bodily experiences, on your thoughts. How comfortable do you feel?

- You may need to move the image forward if you have chosen an experience that will change over time and the image is not unfolding naturally.
- If you can, you can begin to imagine how you'd like the image to be, an ideal experience. Notice what feelings or sensations come with this ideal image or experience.
- Again if this ideal image doesn't feel real, you can imagine colors, sounds, and other details.
- In a few moments, we are going to end this practice; so you might want to bring your awareness to the contact of your legs against the chair.
- And if you've got your eyes closed, open your eyes.

## References

Frijda, N. H. (1986). *The emotions*. Cambridge University Press, Cambridge, UK.

Gross, J. J., & Thompson, R.A. (2007). Emotion regulation: Conceptual foundations. Handbook of emotion regulation (pp. 3–24). New York, NY, USA, Guilford Press.

Magen, E., & Gross, J. J. (2010). *Getting our act together: Toward a general model of self-control. Self-control in society, mind and brain* (pp. 335–353). USA: Oxford University Press.

Mansell, W. (2012). Working with comorbidity in CBT. In W. Dryden, & R. Branch (Eds.), *The CBT handbook*. Los Angeles, CA: SAGE.

Powers, W. T. (2005). *Behavior: The control of perception*. Benchmark Press, New Canaan, CT.

Powers, W. T. (2008). On Emotions and PCT: A Brief Overview. Retrieved from http://www.livingcontrolsystems.com/intro_papers/on

CHAPTER

# 8

# Session 4 Taking Control of the Things Around You

## OVERVIEW

This fourth session focuses on clients' control of their environment; environment referring to work, relationships, housing, etc. It encourages clients to consider which elements of their environment they can, and cannot, control. It also discusses ways of negotiating control within interactions with other people.

The format is the same for all the chapters in Part B. Slides are numbered by session and order; for example, the first slide in this third session would be 4.1, the second slide 4.2. A condensed session plan is provided after the list of all the session materials. Session worksheets are included on the companion website.

## KEY SESSION FOCUS

A unique theme of perceptual control theory (PCT) is that we use our environment to enable us to control our experiences—to get what we want in life. There are many things in our environment that we can change in order to make our world more like we want it to be. However, there are also some things that, objectively, we will have limited control over. Part of our world is other people. This session focuses on helping clients take a wider perspective on their own needs and balancing them with those of people who are important to them.

*Transdiagnostic Group Therapy Training and Implementation*
DOI: https://doi.org/10.1016/B978-0-12-813989-9.00008-7

## OVERALL RATIONALE

The control loop that is described in PCT typically involves the environment, in between action and perception. Our environment provides both the context for us to achieve our goals, and the sources of *disturbances* that may get in the way of our goals. See Box 8.1 for a diagrammatic representation of this. Disturbances can be a very broad range of experiences, such as a traumatic event, difficult relationship(s), a change in boss, or moving cities. Thus, even though the environment is not seen to "trigger" any thoughts or behaviors, as traditionally assumed within cognitive behavioral therapy (CBT), it nevertheless is of integral importance to the process of control, and ultimately, to well-being.

It is important to remember that control in PCT refers to the control of personal experiences, or perceptions, not the control of other people. Yet, because controlling our experiences largely involves acting within the world[1], we can often disturb aspects of our environment that matter to other people. This may lead to a process of "collective control" (McClelland, 2004) or conflict, or both. During collective control people work together to achieve a shared goal, like decorating their family home. Conflict can occur when their desired states of that goal, or their perceptions of where they are in relation to that goal, differ. For example, they may differ on the style they want to decorate the house, or they may differ in their perception of how comfortable they experience a certain choice of furniture. These kinds of conflict are often fully explicit and understandable and are unlikely to lead to prolonged distress. Yet, conflict can also occur as an unintended side effect of two peoples' goals. Some examples may make this clear.

Tom was asked by his wife Amanda to clean the house on his day off from work when he had wanted to relax. He felt annoyed, he thought that he was being "bossed around," and it culminated in a difficult argument. Yet, Amanda explained that her goal was to have a clean house, not to boss her husband around. She had been less aware of her husband's goal of needing to relax, and so conflict ensued. You may remember that we termed this *arbitrary control* (Powers, 1973)—the

[1]Although controlling experiences often involves acting within the world, humans also have access to a rich internal world. Within PCT internal representations and experiences can be utilized without direct contact with the environment. For example, during the goal-focused exposure exercises clients are generally not in direct physical contact with the situation that they are bringing to mind, i.e., they are imagining the situation rather than it originating from external sensory input. This is described as "imagination mode." Importantly, these mental simulations typically entail the attempt to reproduce a similar goal through action within the real environment. "Imagination mode" will be described in more detail in Chapter 10, "Moving Forward: What Gets Me Stuck, What Helps," Part B.

BOX 8.1

## AN EXAMPLE OF A PERCEIVE-COMPARE-ACT FEEDBACK LOOP DEMONSTRATING THE POINT AT WHICH ENVIRONMENTAL FACTORS CAN ACT AS DISTURBANCES

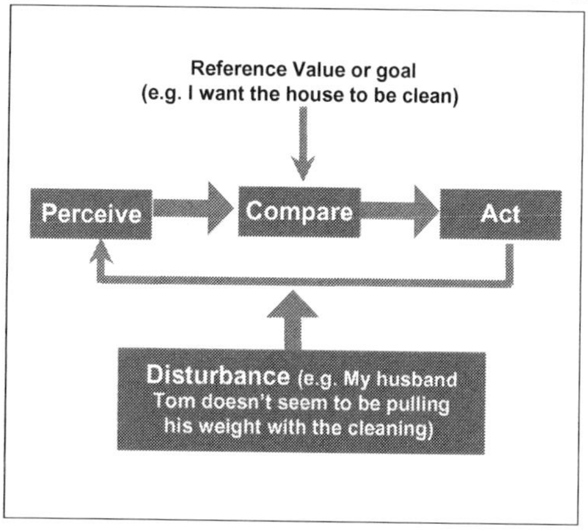


pursuit of a goal without taking into account other important goals that it may conflict with. Arbitrary control can occur between or within individuals. In fact the some of the same processes we discussed earlier can be just as problematic when played out between people, as when they are self-directed. For example, being critical or harsh toward a close friend or family member may be driven by the need to help them (e.g., criticizing their dangerous driving), and yet may clearly interfere with that person's goal of "feeling good about myself". As described in Session 2 (Chapter 6), self-criticism can be functional if it helps meet a goal, such as avoiding dangerous driving, but it can also be experienced as problematic if it conflicts with another goal.

In each case we have discussed it seems clear that the conflict can be better understood when both peoples' goals are brought to the open. Importantly, it appears that it is the higher level, or more fundamental goals, that are most illuminating; it makes sense that we might be critical to a friend who drives badly if we are clear that our goal is to stay safe. So, when there is conflict between two individuals, it is helpful for these individuals to bring awareness to their important (higher level) goals. Individuals can then take steps to clarify their own goals and establish which goals are most important to them. But they will often need to discuss their goal(s) with the other person in order to express it to them and to establish the other person's goal(s). Therefore, in many situations, an important step is letting the other person know that what they are doing is preventing achievement of an important goal. Returning to the example of Tom, Amanda may not realize that Tom is experiencing her suggestions as being dominating, nor that he wants to relax on his day off, for the more fundamental reason that he believes that the chance to relax after a stressful week will make him "a nicer person to be around". In turn, he may not recognize how important it is for Amanda to have a clean house, for the more fundamental reason that she wants to "look like a good mother" when her family visit later that day. We can see that there are potentially many layers of goals behind the more concrete problems (e.g., feeling bossed around) that were raised in the argument.

This process, of clarifying the goals of all those involved, can be applied to a range of interpersonal disputes or conflicts. The second step can often be reaching an agreement that allows those involved to meet their goals, at least to some extent. In reaching compromises it can be helpful to consider if there are any shared higher level goals that agreement can be built upon (McClelland, 1994, 2004). For Tom and Amanda, some possible shared goals are "to have a clean and tidy home," "to be a nice person," with an overall shared goal "it is important that we have a happy relationship." In order to better meet these goals Amanda might agree to be more careful about how, and how often, she expresses suggestions and Tom might agree to treat these as suggestions instead of attempts to boss him around. As interpersonal disputes or conflict always involve more than one person, in many situations it is important to reach an agreement based on shared goals and/or taking into account the goals of the others involved. Therefore this does not require ignoring or suppressing a valued goal for either person. For example, Amanda can take into account that relaxing on his day off is important to Tom, without suppressing her goals to have a clean home and to be a good mother.

As interpersonal conflicts can be very varied, it is important that facilitators maintain a curious approach and avoid unqualified generalizations as much as possible. For example, in the previous paragraph we stated that in *many situations* it is important to reach an agreement based on shared goals. There will be some situations that shared goals cannot be established or that one person's goal is rigidly adhered to (also see next section within this chapter 'Rationale: Is conflict always unhelpful?'). An example of this would be if Tom maintained that he should never do housework. One possibility is that if Tom and Amanda discuss this at another time Tom may see that his goal is undermining another important goal of "having a happy relationship." Thus, again, raising awareness of higher level goals can reduce conflict, this time by reducing rigidity. So the course materials emphasize timing of discussions and suggest that clients consider resuming discussion at another time if an interaction is becoming increasingly confrontational. This can be helpful for two reasons; firstly clients may start to feel out of control if an interaction is escalating. Secondly, when discussions become more confrontational the original and shared goals can seem less important with goals related to "winning the argument" and "getting the point across by any means" given more primacy.

## RATIONALE: IS CONFLICT ALWAYS UNHELPFUL?

The previous section has discussed interpersonal conflict in terms of a problem that needs to be resolved. This is because the course materials are designed to support clients with problems within relationships. However, conflict between individuals is an inevitable part of life. Different people will have different perspectives and goals; consequently these will sometimes conflict. We are suggesting that these conflicts become problematic when they undermine control, that is, when people feel that they cannot achieve the goals that are important to them and feel stuck and distressed. Such conflict will be more problematic when it is enduring, as control will be undermined on an ongoing basis. For example, it was really important to Hayley to have a close relationship with her parents. She had a row with her Dad about another area that was really important to her (how she looked after her children) and they stopped speaking to each other. If her Dad apologized and they came to some understanding regarding the contents of the row, then this would be less likely to undermine her goal to have a close relationship with her parents. However, if this did not happen, and they remained not speaking, she is likely to continue to experience enduring and more problematic loss of control.

There is evidence to support this from the work of Kent McClelland. He developed a computerized simulation of agents controlling the same variable (McClelland, 2004). This provided data regarding what happened when these agents had different reference values for this variable, that is, they had different goals for this variable. Kent also compared this data to data from agents who had the same reference value. The "agents in conflict" had a very similar effect on the variable as when the agents had a shared goal. This may seem counterintuitive but another key aspect was that the "agents in conflict" had to put more and more effort in, in order to control the variable. In a real-life situation this ever-increasing effort would be increasingly demanding and tiring. For example, Leah and Raf argued a lot, Raf starting drinking more alcohol and neither felt happy in their relationship. But they wanted to "keep the family together" until their daughter was older. They stayed together, but still argued and felt frustrated with each other so it took more and more effort to keep the family together.

The key message of this section is very similar to the PCT rationale concerning processes such as worry and self-criticism, and other coping responses—the same process can be both beneficial and problematic. Namely, people in conflict can often achieve their goals despite the conflict, and this maintains the status quo. But even though such enduring conflicts can be tolerated, they often require increasing effort and this can be experienced as fatigue, stress or low mood. If clients are willing to do so, it can still be helpful to bring awareness to these uncomfortable experiences tolerated during conflicts and the higher level goals that underpin these. To return to the example of Raf and Leah, they might realize that while they were able to "keep the family together" despite their arguments and distress, this was not fulfilling the more fundamental goal for why they wanted to keep the family together—to make their daughter happy. For a period of time, until they could understand their own difficulties, it was acceptable to spend time away from the family home. Again, the important message from this section is not around any individual's decisions, but that the solution will come from bringing the goals at the root of any conflict into awareness.

## BEFORE THE SESSION

- Set up the room as described in Chapter 4, How to Use This Book, Part A.
- Print out the relevant session handouts (included on the companion website)
- Bring the relevant materials (listed before the condensed session plan on p. 132).

## SESSION SECTIONS

### Overview of Session

Introduce the theme of the group and give a brief overview of what will be covered during the sessions.

> "There are some things in our environment that we can change and make our world more like we want it to be. There can be some things, about where we live and our environment more generally, that we don't have much control over. But sometimes we can begin to think of ways of making our environment better for us. Naturally, an important part of our world is other people and we will cover some methods that can help us deal with some of the interactions with others we may find tricky."

## Taking Control of Things Around Me: Videos

***Materials:***

Videos of Antony and Cath on "Taking control of things around me" slide 4.2

*Application and practice:* The videos are shown to provide examples of different elements of the environment that were causing stress for previous clients and the ways they found helpful to manage this. The video of Antony illustrates something in his environment that was problematic for him, his work, and this was something that he was able to change. For some of us there may be things in our life we do not like, but that would be difficult to change. For example, work could be problematic, but for contractual or financial reasons it may not be possible to make any instant change.

In Cath's video, she describes some interpersonal issues, avoiding potentially challenging discussions and spending a long time planning what she was going to say. These are areas she had some control over. She describes what helped and did not help with these issues. For example, taking a breath before she explains what the issue is and considering whether the issue is important enough to her to be worth fighting about.

Sometimes clients may question Cath's decision to let the issue she described go, on the basis that they would have addressed it head-on if it happened to them. Although this can be useful point for brief discussion, we are encouraging clients to explore the interpersonal issues that *they themselves* are having problems with and the important goals that relate to these. Consequently, it can be helpful to clarify that the key consideration is whether letting this issue go was in line with Cath's goals. Facilitators can develop this point in order to emphasize the fact that we all have individual goals, which will sometimes be different from another person's. Facilitators can mention that, later in the session, we will focus on the importance of clarifying our own goals and then negotiating these goals in relation to other people's goals.

## How Much Control Do I Have?

***Materials:***

"How much control do I have? Session 4"
Control continuum poster
Pack of large post-it notes
"How much control do I have", slide 4.3

***Take home message***. Control is on a continuum or scale. We have different degrees of control over different things. Given that there could be aspects of our environment that we would like to change, it is important to consider how much control we have over these things. We are talking about environment in the broadest sense, for example, including our relationships, our work, our living arrangements. We are going to consider how much control we have over the aspects of our environment that we want to change. ***Application and practice.*** This is an exercise using the control continuum, similar to the continuum exercise in Session 1. This section begins with the facilitators reading their own examples. They use post-it notes to denote the amount of control they have over an environmental aspect of their life. Ideally this would be a "personal" example, for example, "work deadlines," "relationship with mother-in-law," "when partner does cleaning." It is useful for facilitators to briefly explain why this can cause them problems, and how they have determined their degree of control. For example, "Its really important to me that the house is clean and I find it stressful if my partner does not regularly contribute to the cleaning. I have some control over this as I can discuss it with him, but the level of control is only a six because I don't want to come across as nagging so I don't mention it often."

Give clients "How much control do I have? Session 4" worksheet. This is provided to help clients consider what they want include on postits. Facilitators should explain the purpose of the worksheet. Then ask clients to write down different important and problematic environmental aspects of their life and provide a rating of how much control they have over these. Prompt clients not to include their names. The facilitators collect the post-its (as long as the client is OK with this) and then put the post-it notes on the continuum that is displayed on the wall. The post-its are put up next to the relevant rating, for example, if relationship with mother-in-law is rated as a "4" then the facilitator would stick that post-it next to the number four on the continuum. As each post-it note is placed on the continuum at different locations, this should reveal examples of the full range. Facilitators may decide to add more of their own examples to ensure that the full range is illustrated.

***Discussion and using curious questioning.*** This task is followed by the opportunity for discussion, which may cover a number of areas. A common topic in this session is regarding interpersonal issues, for example, an ongoing conflict/argument. Sometimes these issues have been ongoing for some years and clients feel stuck in interactions that are difficult for them. It can be useful to use curious questioning to explore these issues. However, it is important to try not to get too caught up in detailed accounts of the backstory to the issues. Although it is important that clients are able to clearly identify the problem they are experiencing, PCT would suggest that problematic interactions are likely to remain stuck unless higher level conflicts are brought into awareness. There are a number of ways that greater awareness can be brought to higher level processing through curious questioning. It can be useful to ask about internal or interpersonal processes. An example of an internal process is: "I try to push the bad thoughts down" (i.e., suppression of thoughts) and the clinician could ask questions like: "How far to you push the thoughts?" "What happens when you've pushed the thoughts down?" "Do they go away?" An example of an interpersonal process and questions regarding this is given in Box 8.2. This style of asking questions to bring awareness to higher level processes is reflected in method of levels (MOL) therapy (described in Part A, Chapter 4: How to Use This Book); for a detailed account of how to do MOL see Mansell, Carey, and Tai, 2012.

Some general examples of the kinds of curious questions that can be used are: "What are your thoughts on the number you have chosen?" "Is it higher or lower than you expected?" "Does it sit well with you or do you want it high/lower?" "Can you see what higher or lower would look like?"

## Taking Control With Other People [See companion website for training video]

### *Materials*

Taking control with other people (1)' slide 4.4
"Upward arrow" worksheet
"Taking control with other people (PCA)" slide 4.5
"PCA problem-solving tool" worksheet
"Taking control with other people (2)" slide 4.6
Reference sheet: "Taking control with other people"

*Take home message.* Sometimes it is hard to get the right balance of control in discussions with other people. If you feel like you have no control you might not speak up for yourself, or you might snap or shout at someone to try to get control! Either of these extremes will not get you want in many situations. Clarifying your goals for the discussion, expressing them clearly and allowing other people to express their goals are key steps for taking control.

***Application and practice.* Facilitators describe Step 1, which is detailed on slide 4.4:**

> "A key way to feel in control in interpersonal situations is to know what you want out of the situation and to have this clearly in mind- if you said yes to a request would that fit in with your goals? You can clarify what you want in all kinds of ways: talking the situation through with someone, writing thoughts down etc., using the upward arrow technique and/or PCA problem solving tool."

BOX 8.2

## AN EXAMPLE OF CURIOUS QUESTIONING ABOUT INTERPERSONAL PROCESSES

| | |
|---|---|
| Client: | I'm always arguing with my son about when he gets in at night. |
| Clinician: | Does it bother you when he gets in? |
| Client: | Yes, he always comes home later than we've agreed. |
| Clinician: | Does it bother you more that he is later than agreed, or that he comes in late? |
| Client: | It annoys me more that he doesn't come back when we've agreed. |
| Clinician: | How are you feeling right now, telling me about this? |
| Client: | I feel a bit annoyed, frustrated. |
| Clinician: | What is that feeling like? |
| Client: | Just really wound up, like I'm about to snap. |
| Clinician: | What would happen if you snapped? |
| Client: | I'd yell and him and I might say things I'd regret. |
| Clinician: | How is it going talking about these things right now? Do you want to talk to me a bit more about this after the session? |
| Client: | It's useful to talk through, but I'd prefer to wait until after the session. |

In this example, the facilitator checks out with the client whether they are still comfortable to keep talking even though further questions could have explore the higher level goals involved. This is particularly important given the group context, as clients may not want to discuss in detail in front of others. Also the facilitator has to consider how much the discussion might benefit the other clients and how much material is left to cover.

Within this slide (4.4), facilitators suggest that upward arrow technique can be used to clarify important goals. An upward arrow worksheet with an example is included in Box 8.3 and depicted on slide 4.5. Facilitators explain that in this example Rosie is preparing for a discussion with her romantic partner. Facilitators talk through the example: "This exercise involves starting with an important goal

BOX 8.3

## UPWARD ARROW SLIDE

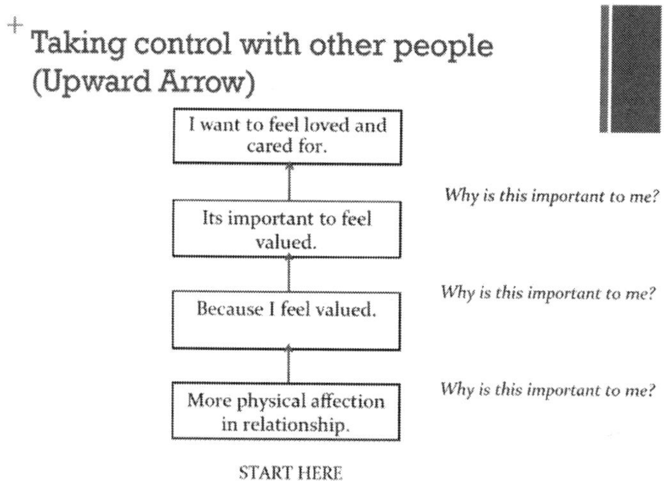


for the discussion, or interpersonal/ environmental problem, e.g. Rosie wrote 'More physical affection in relationship' in the bottom box. Then she asked 'Why is 'More physical affection in relationship' important to me/ why does this help?,' her response was 'Because I feel valued'. She asked 'Why is 'Because I feel valued' important to me/ why does this help?' and her response was 'Its important to feel valued'. She kept on asking this question until she wrote down a really important basic goal in one of the boxes, 'I want to feel loved and cared for' and even though she asked 'why is this important to me?' there was no goal more important than this one."

Explain that, similarly, clients will need to identify an important goal for the discussion, or another interpersonal or environmental problem if they cannot identify a relevant discussion. As in Session 1 when the upward arrow technique was first used, the client will then continue to ask themselves "Why is *X reason/goal* important to me, *or why does it help?"* (the "why is it important question" is usually more useful but occasionally it makes more sense to ask "why it helped"). They keep on asking this question until they write down a really important goal in one of the boxes; for example, I want to be a good parent. These instructions are detailed on the worksheet (see Box 8.4). Facilitators make it clear that clients can make eye contact with the facilitators or gesture

## BOX 8.4

## UPWARD ARROW WORKSHEET

**Upward Arrow: What things are most important to me?**

**Instructions: Upward arrow technique.**

1. Start with the bottom box. Ask yourself:
Why is '*the reason in the bottom box*' important to you/ why does this help?
Put your answer in the box above the bottom one.

2. Each new reason that you write, ask yourself the same questions:
Why is '*X*' important to you/ why does this help?

3. You can stop moving upwards when you end up with a really important basic goal in one of the boxes, e.g. I want to be happy, I want to be a good parent.

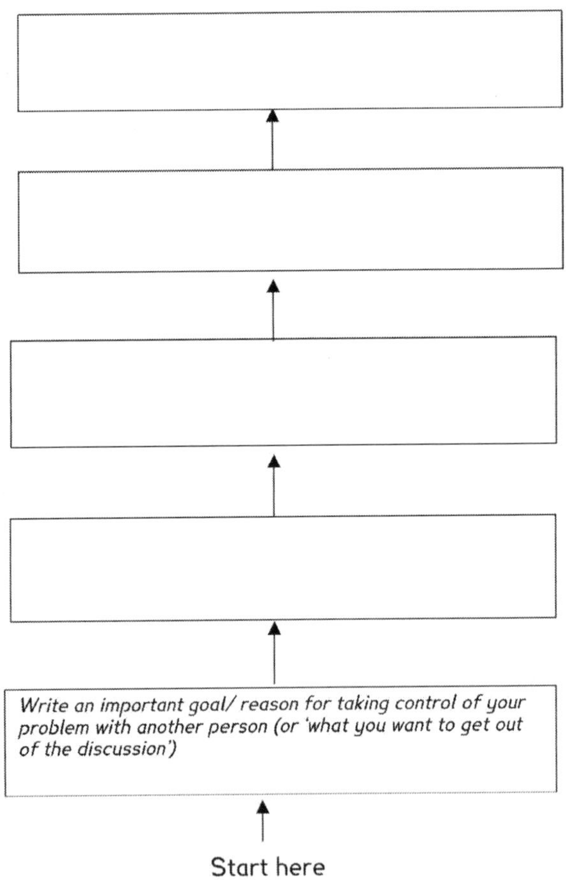

them over if they want to clarify something. Occasionally clients will start with a higher level goal. If this arises the technique can be used to clarify what this means for the client; for example, what does being a good parent look like? This involves asking the question "what does that look like, or what does that mean in practice?", instead of "Why is *X reason/goal* important to me?"

The PCA tool can be used to further clarify goals and identify if any conflicted goals are blocking achievement of important goals. Facilitators provide a personal example of the PCA tool (the relevant slide for the PCA section is 4.6). They then ask clients to complete the PCA tool to clarify their problems and goals related to an interpersonal issue or conflict. If clients cannot think of an interpersonal issue then they could use the PCA tool to work through other problems and goals related to their environment (regarding housing, work or other areas). Following the exercise facilitators can use curious questioning to check understanding of the tool, for example, "how did you find doing that?" "Did it make sense?" "Did you have any problems filling in any sections?" Other curious questions that can be used as appropriate are: "Was the actions you thought of expected/unexpected?" "Did any solutions come to mind?" "Is there anything in the way of you achieving this other goal (conflicting goal)?" "Did you think of anything additional after recognizing the other goal?"

**Facilitators talk through Steps 2 and 3 (detailed on slide 4.7 and elaborated below):**

> "Once you've clarified your goals often the next step is discussing these with the other person (or people) involved. Before going into the discussion, it can be worth thinking about how much you are willing to compromise and this will depend on what is being asked of you. During the discussion it is useful to make sure you are clear what the other person is asking of you and to try to clarify what their goals are. Sometimes you may find that you share goals with the other person and this can be used to build a compromise that works well for both of you.
>
> If you find yourself in an interpersonal situation that is becoming increasingly confrontational: check how the situation is for you (how comfortable/ uncomfortable), have you said what you want to, would it be worth suggesting dropping the subject and coming back to it?"

Facilitators can make suggestions regarding dealing with the "aftermath" of challenging interactions (described in more detail on "Taking control with other people" reference sheet):

> "For some of us, clearly expressing what we want can be a challenge and this can be even more challenging with certain people. If a discussion or interaction has been challenging it is important to look after ourselves. Try to make a deal with yourself to take a break before you think about the discussion you have had. Often we can want to think about the discussion repeatedly, it is worth considering how helpful this will be."

If covered in Session 2 (Chapter 6), facilitators can suggest that clients watch out for the "self-critical voice/negative thought monster".

## Taking Control With Other People: Awareness of Important Goals/Values [See companion website for training video]

***Materials:***

"An example..." slide 4.8
"Another example..." slide 4.9
"Another example... (2)" slide 4.10
"Another example... (3)" slide 4.11

***Take home message.*** During discussions or interactions with others, it can be useful to consider if there are any shared goals. Shared goals can help reach agreements that suit everyone. Focusing on shared goals can also make it less likely that we get lost in the details of the argument, for example, getting caught up in "scoring points" against the other person. Another useful way to prevent getting too caught up in the argument is keeping in mind the goals that are really important to us and reflecting on whether the argument is helping us meet these.

***Application and practice.*** There are a number of slides that illustrate examples of discussions in which one or both parties used shared goals to come to an agreement.

The facilitators talk through the "speech bubble slides." The majority of these slides are set up so that the speech bubble appear sequentially; for example, the first slide appears empty and clicking forward makes the first speech bubble appear ("You never listen") and clicking forward again makes the second speech bubble appear ("I do listen!!").

Facilitators introduce the first example (see Box 8.5) by mentioning that it depicts quite a short argument. If appropriate facilitators can joke that this is how all their disagreements go, that is, alluding to the fact that some discussions are not resolved as quickly as this. They then go through the speech bubbles depicted on slide 4.8 (Box 8.5). It can make it more entertaining if the facilitator(s) emphasize the argumentative tone of voice of the friends depicted in the slides. As a summary, the facilitator mentions that the friends realize that they have an important shared goal of wanting to spend time together and are able to agree a way that is convenient for both of them to meet this goal.

The second example depicts another discussion- one that has become more argumentative (See Box 8.6). Facilitators talk through the example on slide 4.9 that depicts this argument. They then mention that during

BOX 8.5

## FIRST EXAMPLE SLIDES FROM TAKING CONTROL WITH OTHER PEOPLE: AWARENESS OF IMPORTANT GOALS/ VALUES

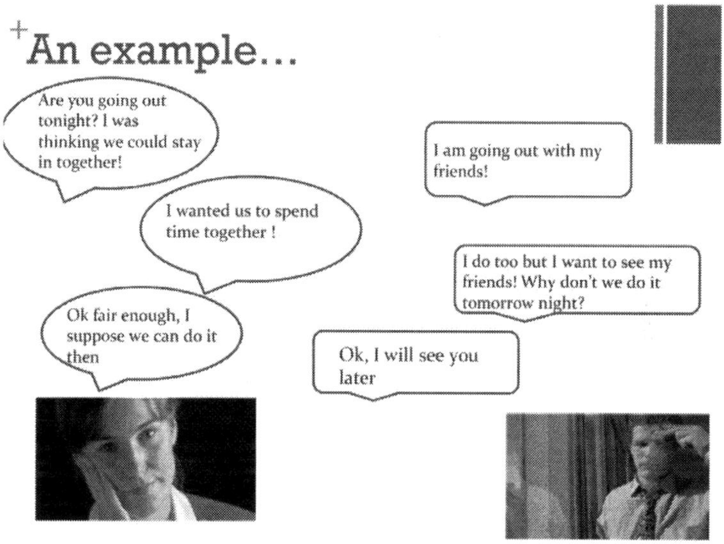


the course of the argument one of the couple reflects and becomes aware of their most important goal. Her reflective process is depicted in slide 4.10 (Box 8.7). As she reflects she realizes that the relationship is more important to her than the issue they are arguing about. She says "I don't think this argument is worth fighting about" and they are able to reach an agreement. In this example she realizes the issue that she is raising is not as important as the positive relationship she has with her partner, which is really important (Box 8.8).

As demonstrated within these examples, considering both shared and higher level, important goals can help meet both parties' goals. Clearly relationships can be complex and it is common that clients need to discuss their own experiences to consider how these principles could be relevant to them. Examples of curious questioning include: "Do you notice any key themes?" "How does this example sit with you?" "What are your thoughts on how conflict was dealt with?" "What's getting in

BOX 8.6

**SECOND EXAMPLE SLIDES FROM TAKING CONTROL WITH OTHER PEOPLE: AWARENESS OF IMPORTANT GOALS/ VALUES. THIS IS THE FIRST SLIDE OF THREE IN THIS EXAMPLE**

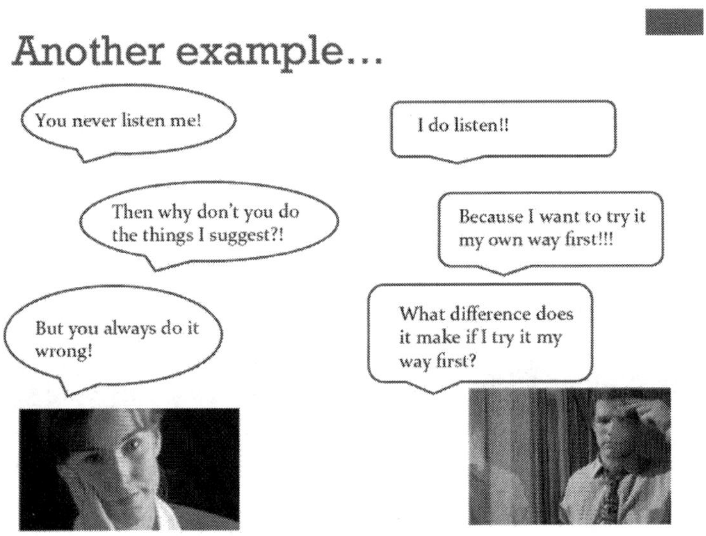


the way of dealing with conflict?" "What does it mean for you to deal with conflict?" "What can you do when another person has different views/beliefs on conflict?" "Any different ideas come up for you?" As ever these questions are given as examples, the facilitator will need to respond appropriately to the flow of discussion and clients' individual situations.

## Taking Control in Imagination

***Materials:***

Reference slide: "Choosing an experience I want to take control of" (4.12)
"Choosing an experience I want to take control of" worksheet
Facilitator prompt sheets: "Session 4- guided exposure in imagination" and "Guided exposure in imagination"

BOX 8.7

## SECOND EXAMPLE SLIDES FROM TAKING CONTROL WITH OTHER PEOPLE: AWARENESS OF IMPORTANT GOALS/ VALUES. THIS IS THE SECOND SLIDE OF THREE IN THIS EXAMPLE

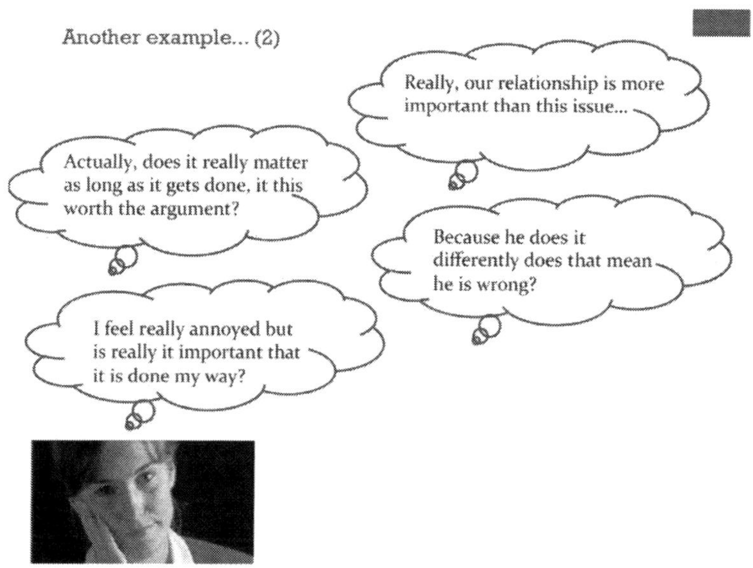


***Take home message and link to previous sections.*** There are a number of ways of taking control in problematic situations with other people, such as speaking to the other person. However, we can be held back by concern that this will be uncomfortable or concern that we will not be able to express ourselves clearly. We can begin to take control of these concerns by bringing such situations to mind and seeing how they unfold in our minds eye. Bringing such situations to mind can also change our perspective on them.

***Application and practice.*** During this version of the taking control in imagination exercise we are encouraging clients to bring an interpersonal issue to mind, this can be an issue at home, at work, with family or with friends. Use the slide "Choosing an experience I want to take control of" (depicted in Box 8.9) to encourage clients to think of an interpersonal issue that is preventing them from achieving important goals.

BOX 8.8

**SECOND EXAMPLE SLIDES FROM TAKING CONTROL WITH OTHER PEOPLE: AWARENESS OF IMPORTANT GOALS/ VALUES. THIS IS THE THIRD SLIDE OF THREE IN THIS EXAMPLE**

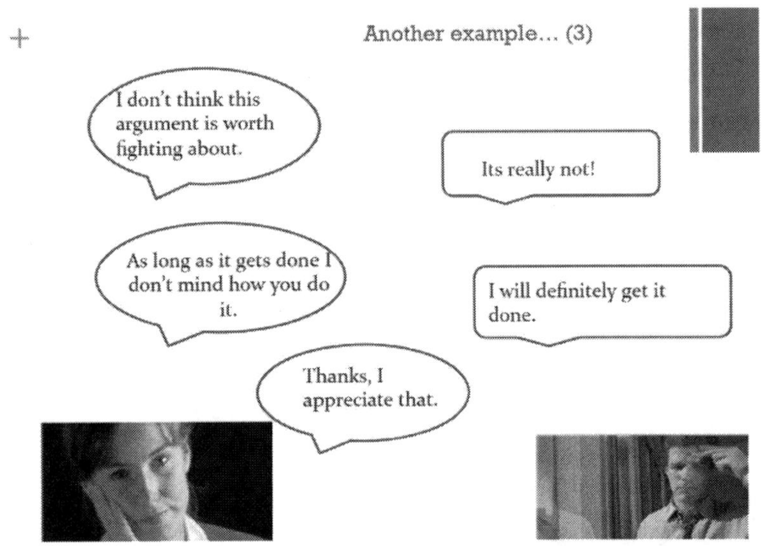


At this point facilitators can ask the group if they would prefer to focus on a general problem rather than an interpersonal one. If a number of clients say they would prefer a general problem then the facilitator can use the procedure from the previous session; however, facilitators should make it clear that any client who wants to focus on an interpersonal issue can still do so.

Toward the bottom of the "Choosing an experience I want to take control of" worksheet there is a space for clients to fill-in why it might help them to face the experience/situation they have chosen, that is, the important goal that is being blocked. However, even when they are choosing the experience/situation that they want to take control of is important to encourage clients to consider what they ultimately want out of going through this situation in their minds eye? They may want to refer back to the upward arrow technique completed earlier in the

### BOX 8.9

## EXAMPLE OF "CHOOSING AN EXPERIENCE I WANT TO TAKE CONTROL OF" SLIDE

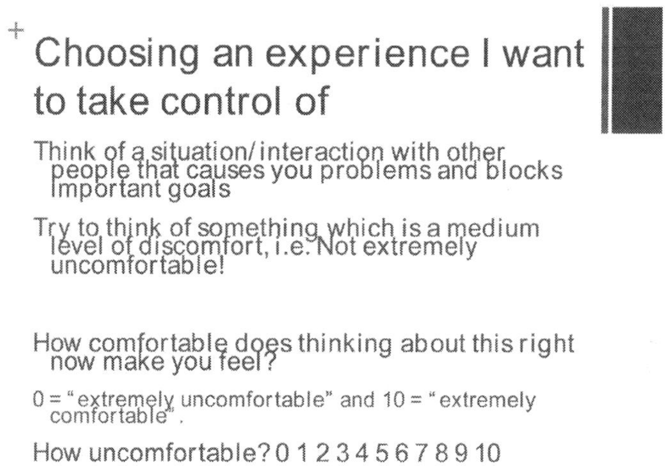


session to identify really important goals. The experience chosen should be an issue/experience that is around a 4/5 level of discomfort, or "medium level" of discomfort. It is worth reminding clients that the important thing is that the experience is not so challenging and uncomfortable that it will be too distressing or overwhelming for them to stay with it.

Lead through the guided exposure exercise using the relevant prompt sheet. Mostly this will be the "Session 4- guided exposure in imagination prompts", but if the group has expressed a preference for focusing on general problems the facilitator should use the "Guided exposure in imagination prompts" (provided on p. 134).

If interpersonal issues were addressed during this exercise, facilitators can emphasize the following (after the exercise): "If you brought to mind a challenging interpersonal situation and feel a bit upset or agitated, then you could make a deal with yourself to give yourself a break before thinking about it. It may help to consider how much to be gained from dwelling on what has happened and you may want to do something that you enjoy or find relaxing so that you are less likely to dwell on the issue."

## Optional: Awareness Exercise

***Materials:***

Body awareness prompts

***Take home message and link to previous sections.*** Awareness techniques can help us notice our emotions and experiences without feeling that we have to change them. Sometimes we cannot change our environment, but bringing awareness to an environmental situation/experience can sometimes change our perspective on such situations/experiences.

***Application and practice.*** Ask participants to pay attention to sensations in body (they can close their eyes if they want), then ask what they noticed. Lead participants through imagining a metaphor, bringing the image to mind as part of the awareness practice (see Appendix F for examples of metaphors). The metaphor models one way of interacting with thoughts and experiences, by noticing and letting thoughts go past.

## Thinking About the Week Ahead

***Materials:***

Reference slide: "Thinking about the week ahead" (4.13)

"Thinking about the week ahead" worksheet

***Take home message.*** Some of the things that cause us problems are in our environment. When we have control over these things we may be able to change them. But sometimes we cannot change these external things and may have to change how we interact with them instead.

***Application and practice.*** Encourage participants to fill in the "Thinking about the week ahead" worksheet. Encourage them to include specific goals and ways of remembering these as appropriate.

# MATERIALS REQUIRED

## Worksheets required:

How much control do I have

Upward arrow

PCA problem solving

Taking control with other people

Choosing an experience I want to take control of

Thinking about the week ahead

**Facilitator prompts required:**

Body awareness prompts
Session 4- guided exposure in imagination prompts
Guided exposure in imagination prompts

**Other materials required:**

Post its
Control continuum
Pens
Projector to show PowerPoint slides and videos
Laptop (to use with projector)
Speakers
PowerPoint presentation
Clinical measures

## DON'T FORGET

- Use curious questioning to help clients develop understanding.
- Try to let *take home messages* emerge from client comments/ discussion.
- When responding to the group, try to check out what is best for individual group members to enable them to maintain control.
- Where appropriate link each session to previous sessions or session sections.

## END OF CHAPTER QUIZ

In order for you to check what you have taken in, we have devised a short quiz. We suggest giving each question a go before checking the answers!

How can the environment influence our level of control from a PCT perspective? (p. 114)
Give a personal example of something in the environment that you feel you have some control over (e.g., using a rating and description as in the continuum exercise) (p. 119–120)
Explain the use of the upward arrow tool in interpersonal situations (p. 122–123)
Explain the take home message for the "speech bubble" slides (p. 126)

# CONDENSED SESSION PLAN: SESSION 4

| | |
|---|---|
| Measures | Give clients the clinical measures prior to the session |
| Theme<br>*3 min* | Introduce the theme of the session |
| Taking control of things around me: Videos *5 min* | Antony and Cath discussing environmental or interpersonal issues |
| How much control do I have?<br>*5–10 min* | Continuum of control exercise |
| Taking control with other people<br>*15–20 min* | Facilitators go through three steps of:<br>**1.** Clarifying most important goals using "Upward Arrow" worksheet<br>Further clarify goals and identify conflicts: PCA problem-solving tool<br>**2.** Deciding how much willing to compromise<br>**3.** Expressing what want clearly and assertively<br>Briefly discuss "aftermath" of challenging interactions<br>***SHOULD BE AT LEAST HALFWAY THROUGH*** |
| Taking control with other people: Awareness of important goals/values<br>*5 min* | Talk through the two examples of discussions/arguments depicted in "speech bubbles" on the slides. Draw out the key themes of developing shared goals (example 1) and keeping in mind key goals (example 2) |
| Taking control in imagination<br>*10–15 min* | Facilitate clients to identify a manageable experience. Lead through exercise using "Session 4- guided exposure in imagination prompts" (or "Guided exposure in imagination prompts") |
| ***Optional***: How to take control: Awareness exercise *5–10 min* | Includes:<br>– Brief introduction: Bringing awareness to a problematic environmental situation/experience, which we cannot change, can alter our perspective<br>– Body awareness exercise (use body awareness prompts) |
| Thinking about the week ahead<br>*2–5 min* | Brief summary of the session<br>Clients identify what they want to do at home |
| Evaluation form and additional sheets | Give participants the sessional evaluation form. Advise participants that there are some information sheets that they can take if they want to on "Work colleagues and employers" |

## SESSION 4: GUIDED EXPOSURE IN IMAGINATION PROMPTS

Lead through awareness exercise for 3 min. Note: the below are prompts which are not intended to be read out like a list but intended to be "dropped into" the practice at appropriate intervals; use your discretion as to whether all the prompts are appropriate.

- As before you may want to close your eyes.
- Can you bring an image of the situation to mind.
- How vivid and real does it feel? If it doesn't feel very vivid you may want to try and imagine sounds or smells if appropriate, or focus on the colors and details within the image.
- Try to say what you need to say in a clear and assertive way.
- Notice what effect imagining this situation is having on you, on your bodily experiences, on your thoughts. How comfortable do you feel?
- How is the other person reacting, what are they saying?
- Again if the image to doesn't feel real you can imagine colors, sounds, and other details.
- Have you said what you needed to say? Is it helpful to continue the discussion at this time?
- If you are feeling upset after the discussion, give yourself a chance to calm down before you think about it, for example, doing something you enjoy.
- Consider how much to be gained from dwelling on, or replaying, what has happened.

## GUIDED EXPOSURE IN IMAGINATION PROMPTS

Lead through awareness exercise for 3 min. Note: The below are prompts which are not intended to be read out like a list but intended to be "dropped into" the practice at appropriate intervals.

- As before you may want to close your eyes.
- Can you bring an image of the situation or experience to mind?
- If it is difficult to bring an image to mind, you may be able to get a sense of how you'd feel or you could even try bringing a memory to mind.
- How vivid and real does it feel? If it doesn't feel very vivid you may want to try and imagine sounds or smells if appropriate, or focus on the colors and details within the image.
- Notice what effect imagining this experience is having on you, on your bodily experiences, on your thoughts. How comfortable do you feel?

- You may need to move the image forward if you have chosen an experience that will change over time and the image is not unfolding naturally.
- If you can you can begin to imagine how you'd like the image to be, an ideal experience. Notice what feelings or sensations come with this ideal image or experience.
- Again if this ideal image doesn't feel real you can imagine colors, sounds and other details.
- In a few moments we are going to end this practice, so you might want to bring your awareness to the contact of your legs against the chair.

And if you've got your eyes closed, open your eyes.

## References

Mansell, W., Carey, T. A., & Tai, S. J. (2012). *A transdiagnostic approach to CBT using method of levels therapy: Distinctive features*. New York: Routledge.

Mc Clelland, K. (1994). Perceptual control and social power. *Sociological Perspectives, 37*(4), 461–496. Available from https://doi.org/10.2307/1389276.

Mc Clelland, K. (2004). The collective control of perceptions: constructing order from conflict. *International Journal of Human-Computer Studies, 60*(1), 65–99. Available from https://doi.org/10.1016/j.ijhcs.2003.08.003.

Powers, W. T. (1973). Behavior: the Control of Perception. Chicago, Il: Aldine.

CHAPTER

# 9

# Session 5 Building on Strengths, Qualities, and Resources

## OVERVIEW

This fifth session focuses on encouraging clients to identify and use the available personal qualities and resources that they have. The session covers a range of resources from everyday supports and achievements to personal qualities or strengths. It prompts clients to consider their resources and strengths in broad terms and reflects the fact that different individuals will have very different resources available to them.

The format will be the same for all the chapters in Part B. Slides are numbered by session and order; for example, the first slide in this session would be 5.1, the second slide 5.2. A condensed session plan is provided after the list of all the session materials. Session worksheets are included on the companion website.

## KEY SESSION FOCUS

The focus of the session is to encourage clients to recall the strengths, qualities, and resources they have, especially at times when things are difficult for them. These are the things inside themselves and within their social world that will help them take control of their lives.

*Transdiagnostic Group Therapy Training and Implementation*
DOI: https://doi.org/10.1016/B978-0-12-813989-9.00009-9

## OVERALL RATIONALE

The strengths, qualities, and resources that clients have can support them with different problems, which they have varying levels of control over. For example, some clients may feel totally out of control and be experiencing an overwhelming conflict; other clients may have regained some control. An example of a client who was feeling totally out of control is Clara. She was suffering from bouts of acute anxiety, could not identify a clear reason for this and felt that she was "going mad." She was beginning to struggle doing everyday tasks and had to take some time off her job. Malid, however, had regained some control; he was aware that one of the reasons he was having problems was a recent romantic relationship that had ended badly and was able to do many of his normal activities. There were times, e.g., when he was at work, when he could mostly get on with what he was doing without thinking about problems within romantic relationships. But outside of work, this often dominated his thinking. For both of these clients, it could be beneficial to consider the strengths, qualities, and resources available to them.

The perceptual control theory (PCT) perspective gives us a framework to understand what maybe meant by strengths, qualities, and resources. PCT states that we are fundamentally purposeful; life is a process of getting our experiences to match with how we want them to be. We organize these desired experiences into a hierarchy, and those at the top are deeper and more fundamental. Yet, they can often lie outside awareness. By asking certain questions, we can help people to bring these to the surface—for example, to be a kind person; to be strong for my family. The better we can bring these goals into our perception—for example, through rich imagery—the better we can identify when we are using our strengths, qualities, and resources to achieve them. What we describe as strengths and qualities are likely to be the lower level systems that we use to achieve our higher level goals, such as an ability to listen carefully in order to help other people. The resources may include important aspects of our environment, that "close the loop" between our actions and our experiences (called the "feedback function" or "feedback pathway")—for example, to fulfill the goal of "being connected with other people," we need to spend time with a person who shares a similar need. Thus, we can see that from a PCT perspective, certain features of our environment are essential to have control over our lives; the environment is not a "trigger" for a response, it is a component of the continuously active "loops" between us and the world.

Returning to the clinical examples, Clara felt overwhelmed and out of control, and so it is important that she could feel that she had enough control to begin to tackle her problems. When people are highly distressed, anxious, or feel that "their world is crashing down around them", then it can be difficult to process their problems, as these can feel overwhelming or unmanageable in other ways. When people are experiencing ongoing difficulties, certain important goals can be undermined; for example, individuals may start to doubt that they can be a strong or capable person, or that are able to be a good partner or friend. Therefore, it can be beneficial for clients to bring to mind the things that they can do, supportive people in their lives and other broad qualities and resources, in order to support them to process/address difficulties. One of the ways in which this is encouraged is using a "strengths, qualities, and resources" checklist, which lists everyday qualities and resources for clients to endorse. This checklist includes items such as "I have taken care of myself in some way (e.g., bath, shower, eating nice food)," "I have learned something in a book, magazine, newspaper, internet, or on the television," and "I have been honest with myself about how I feel." Completing the checklist can also help people to identify that they are achieving certain goals, such as caring for themselves or learning new things. Other exercises that promote identification and utilization of strengths and resources include the client identifying their "top 5 strengths and resources" and creating a supportive image that can help them bring personally important strengths and qualities to mind. Studies have shown that perceptions of well-being are enhanced when personal goals are achieved (Brunstein, 1993; Sheldon & Kasser, 1995) and that focusing on personal strengths increases positive affect, when compared to a control condition and an exercise focused on gratitude (Sheldon & Lyubomirsky, 2006).

For Malid and other clients who have some control, and have an initial awareness of the problem and related conflict(s), these exercises could still be useful. By considering the resources and strengths that they have, clients could become aware of any blocks (or conflicts) that are preventing them from fully accessing their resources. Malid realized that he never dwelt on relationships that have been generally happy and harmonious, and that he was only dwelling on his recent relationship difficulties because he felt he needed to work out why that one relationship "went wrong." After considering his strengths and resources, he realized that this way of thinking had prevented him from recognizing his strengths within relationships and ultimately prevented him from moving toward his goal of "building a new relationship." Other examples of conflicting goals/reference values that could prevent clients from utilizing their resources include not talking to friends because they "do not want to burden them," not spending money on activities they enjoy because they have a reference value that "spending money on myself is wasteful," or not making time for themselves because "making time for myself is selfish."

In addition to this, the strengths and qualities described by people often represent values that are important to them. Identifying the strength "I'm a kind person" implies that being kind is important to the person. Goals, such as "it's important to be kind," and "I want to be a good friend," can be described as self-concept goals and are important higher level reference values. Given the importance of such reference values, difficulties and distress arise when another reference value remains in conflict with a self-concept reference value; for example, "I must be strong" vs "I am weak and inadequate" (Tai, 2009). It is possible that the belief in personal weakness is in turn driven by the need to depend on other people, and it fulfills the goal of being close to them. By becoming more aware of the strengths and values that are important to them, clients may also become more aware of important, higher level conflicts.

If clients have largely resolved the problems and conflicts that they were facing, the content of this session could still be useful for them. By drawing on their strengths and resources, this can help them pursue the goals that are really important to them and to build new ones for the future (Niemiec, 2013). For example, Sian had become aware that she had a conflict between feeling she had to spend all her time caring for her husband and making time for herself. However, she had devoted so much time and energy caring for him that she found it hard to decide what to do when she made time for herself. Through reflecting on her strengths and resources, it occurred to her that she had previously enjoyed creative activities and had a good eye for color, and she began to make cards. Further, this session is the penultimate session of the Course, and it is useful for clients to consider the strengths and resources they can draw on once the Course is over. Although the final session gives clients the opportunity to reflect on what they are taking from the Course, Session 5 focuses on strengths and resources in much more detail.

## BEFORE THE SESSION

- Set up the room as described in Chapter 4, How to Use This Book, Part A.
- Print out the relevant session handouts (included on the companion website).
- Bring the relevant materials (listed before the condensed session plan on p. 146).

# SESSION SECTIONS

## Overview of Session

### *Materials*

Reference slide: "Strengths, qualities, and resources" (5.2)

Introduce the theme of the group and give a brief overview of what will be covered during the session.

> It is easy to forget the strengths, opportunities and resources we have; sometimes these can seem trivial to us. An example of an opportunity is a time when can read handouts from this Course, an example of a strength is 'determination' and an example of a resource is 'people around you that might be able to help'. Our strengths and resources can help us to take control of our problems.

One way to think about the importance of our strengths and resources is using a metaphor of a tree:

> You can think of taking control of your problems like nurturing a young tree, the tree needs resources such as water, sun light and nutrients, to grow. These resources are like the resources you all have which will help you take control. The tree will still experience harsh weather, wind and rain, in the same way you will face threats and challenges at times. However, when the tree is given the resources it needs gradually over time its strength and ability to weather the storms will increase.
>
> These sessions are also designed to provide you with additional resources.

## Thinking About Strengths and Resources Broadly: Video

### *Materials*

Slide: "My resources" (5.3)
*Application and practice:* Antony talks about his son helping him indirectly, i.e., by being a person Antony valued and "derived" strength from. His son was not aware of this, but Antony was able to draw on this relationship to keep motivated. This is an example of the fact that the resources available to us can be broad. As ever, it is useful to give clients the opportunity to comment or ask questions if they want. For example, clients may relate to Antony's relationship with his son directly, i.e., they have people in their lives that they "draw" strength from; or they may identify other broad resources, such as really enjoying listening to music/watching TV, and finding this helps give them a break from the problems they are experiencing.
*Take home message:* The strengths and resources that we can draw on can be broader than we think. Sometimes, we might not realize the

strengths that we have and the things, or people, in our lives that we draw inspiration from. In this session, we will look at some ways of bringing any general strengths and resources that you have to mind.

## "Strengths, Qualities, and Resources" Checklist

### *Materials*

Reference slide: "Strengths, resources checklist" (5.4)
Worksheets: "Strengths, qualities, and resources" and "Checklist of Strengths, qualities, and resources"
*Take home message:* Particularly when we are experiencing problems, it can be really hard to think of our strengths and resources. It can be easy to dismiss the things that we do even though they are of value. This puts us in a difficult situation as we need to draw on our strengths and resources to take control of the problems we are experiencing.
*Application and practice:* Facilitators ask client to fill in the "strengths, qualities, and resources" checklist. Facilitators can use the take home message to explain why it is important to consider the beneficial everyday things we do. Facilitators should mention that there are two versions, on pages 1 and 2 of the session worksheets, and explain that clients can choose which one they use.

Some examples of curious questions are as follows: "How was that exercise for you?", "Have you noticed any strengths or qualities that you weren't expecting?", "Have you noticed any you've not done in a while?", "Did you notice anything you want to change?"

## Recognizing My Personal Qualities: Videos

### *Materials*

Slide: "Recognizing my personal qualities" (5.5)
*Application and practice:* In both the videos, Sarah and Cath describe greater recognition of their personal qualities and strengths. Sarah talks about recognizing how strong she is given what she has dealt with. She also mentions that she has noticed that she is more patient with herself and gets less annoyed with herself. Cath talks about recognizing and appreciating her personal qualities more generally. The specific personal qualities she describes are an organizing quality and also that she is brilliant at buying presents.
*Take home message:* It can be helpful to recognize personal qualities; including quite idiosyncratic qualities, such as present-buying skills! These qualities can help us take control of our problems and recognize when we have achieved something important to us.

Sometimes, we can become more aware of our personal qualities when we are experiencing difficulties, like Sarah became more aware of how strong she is.

## Top 5 Strengths, Qualities, and Resources

### *Materials*

Worksheet: "Top 5 Strengths, qualities and resources"
*Link to previous section and take home message:* Both Sarah and Cath talked about recognizing and appreciating their own positive qualities. Recognizing and appreciating our own positive qualities or strengths are particularly hard to do! We often get the message from society etc. that thinking about our positive qualities is a bit big headed when in fact it is a vital way of maintaining our confidence and taking control of problems.
*Application and practice:* Facilitators ask clients to fill in the "Top 5 Strengths, qualities, and resources" worksheet. Suggest that clients mostly try to think of personal qualities, e.g., I'm a kind person, good listener, help people out, or have a good sense of humor. It can be useful to provide the below suggestion once clients start completing the worksheet:

> One thing that can help if you're finding it hard to think of your strengths and qualities is thinking about what a good friend or family member, or someone else in your life that you know appreciates you, would say about you.

Some potential curious questions that can be used as appropriate are as follows: "How did you find that?", "Was it easier/harder than you expected?", "Any strengths that were unexpected?", "How was it to recognize/think about your own qualities?", "Was it useful?"

## How to Take Control: Developing a Supportive Image [See companion website for training video]

### *Materials*

Reference slide: "Developing a supportive image" (5.6)
*Link to previous sessions and take home message:* In this section, we are going to develop a supportive image. *Facilitators can mention that this image could be a counterpart to the critical/negative monster image developed in Session 2, if they used this technique. The supportive image does not replace the critical/negative monster image but is likely to serve a different role.* We talked about how hard it is to keep in mind our positive qualities and strengths when we are experiencing

difficulties. The supportive image can help us bring these strengths and qualities to mind. Alternatively, we can use the supportive image as a resource to meet our important goals in other ways. For example, if you want to be less critical of yourself, so you can achieve the goal of "feeling confident," you could develop an image that expresses nonjudgmental warmth, or if you want strength to address a difficult interpersonal situation that is blocking your goals, then you could develop an image that makes you feel strong or courageous.

*Application and practice:* Facilitators suggest that clients avoid using an actual person and suggest that they can use a fantasy/fictional character or spiritual presence instead. Clients can also use a place or even a memory as their image. Facilitator should give an example, such as "I bring to mind a beach with golden sand, blue-green sea, and warm sun, and the quality I get from this is relaxation. So I sometimes bring it to mind at times when I'm feeling stressed and I need to focus."

Facilitators explain the worksheet. The supportive image could include the following qualities:

- Soothing
- Strong
- Accepting nonjudgmental
- Warm

The quality clients chose to promote in their image would depend very much on what they want to get from the image. To consider this, clients can ask themselves

- What do I need this supportive image to be like?
- What characteristics or qualities does my supportive image need to have?

To help them develop the image further they can notice the details of and responses to the image, such as:

- Do you associate a particular smell with the image?
- Are they saying anything, if so, what is their tone of voice?
- What do you feel in your body in response?

Facilitators then ask clients to fill in their responses on the worksheet. As ever, facilitators should make it clear that clients can make eye contact with them or gesture them over if they want to clarify something. Sometimes, clients want to discuss the image that they have developed, but this is not always the case—possibly because the image can express something quite personal to the client. Some examples of curious questions are as follows: "Did your image incorporate the qualities you wanted?", "Did your experience change when you introduced your supportive image?", "Did you find it useful to develop an image?"

## How to Take Control: Compassionate Awareness Exercise

### *Materials*

"Compassionate awareness" facilitator prompts

*Take home message:* Sometimes, one of the blocks to us taking control is that we feel that we cannot meet our goals. This could be for all sorts of reasons, such as feeling like a failure, mistakes reducing confidence, and feeling undermined by the problems being faced. This exercise helps us to keep our strengths in mind and work with such issues in order to meet the goals that are really important to us.

*Application and practice:* Lead through compassionate awareness (see prompts: compassionate awareness on p. 148). Before facilitators start, please mention to participants that during the practice they will encourage clients to bring to mind a recent mistake, or something they felt bad about. Give clients a few seconds to think about what they might use. As with any of the visualisations, there maybe aspects that are difficult for certain people to connect with; it is important to let clients know that they can keep coming back to the facilitators prompts even if they can't visualise easily or don't strongly connect with a particular aspect.

This practice also includes bringing the supportive image, and any strengths identified, to mind. As with the awareness exercises, the prompts should not be read out like a list but mentioned with appropriate amounts of space between each prompt. If facilitators are not familiar with such practices, it is recommended that they listen to the self-compassion/loving-kindness meditation that can be downloaded from http://www.self-compassion.org/guided-self-compassion-meditations-mp3.html. This practice is somewhat similar to the one within the session and so provides an example of the general style that is appropriate.

## Thinking About the Week Ahead

### *Materials*

Reference slide: "Thinking about the week ahead" (5.7)

"Thinking about the week ahead" worksheet

*Take home message:* Like our goals, our strengths and resources are important in taking control of our problems. It can be especially important to remember these strengths and resources during times of difficulty and stress.

*Application and practice:* Encourage participants to fill in the "Thinking about the week ahead" worksheet. Encourage them to include specific goals and ways of remembering these as appropriate. For example, one client in a previous Course said that she found it helpful to put the "Strengths, qualities, and resources" checklist on her fridge as this helped her keep this in mind.

## MATERIALS REQUIRED

**Worksheets required:**

Strengths, qualities, and resources
Checklist of Strengths, qualities, and resources
Top 5 Strengths, qualities, and resources
Developing a supportive image
Thinking about the week ahead

**Facilitator prompts required:**

Compassionate awareness

**Other materials required:**

Pens
Projector to show PowerPoint slides and videos
Laptop (to use with projector)
Speakers
PowerPoint presentation
Clinical measures

## END OF CHAPTER QUIZ

In order for you to check what you have taken in, we have devised a short quiz. We suggest giving each question a go before checking the answers!

Why is it important to look at strengths, qualities, and resources? (p. 138–139, 141)
Explain what a supportive image is. (p. 143–144)
What is the rationale for using a compassionate awareness exercise that incorporates a supportive image? (p. 145)

# CONDENSED SESSION PLAN: SESSION 5

| | |
|---|---|
| Measures | Give clients the clinical measures prior to the session |
| Theme/overview<br>*5 min* | Introduce the theme of the session, including the tree metaphor |
| Thinking about strengths and resources broadly: Video<br>*3 min* | Antony describes that he "drew strength" from his son |
| Strengths, qualities and resources checklist<br>*5–10 min* | Facilitators ask clients to complete one of the versions of the "strengths, qualities, and resources checklist" |
| Recognizing my personal qualities: Videos<br>*3 min* | Sarah and Cath discuss recognizing their strengths and personal qualities |
| Top 5 Strengths, qualities and resources<br>*5–10 min* | Facilitators ask clients to complete their top 5 strengths and resources on the worksheet<br>*SHOULD BE AT LEAST HALFWAY THROUGH* |
| How to take control: developing a supportive image<br>*5–10 min* | Includes<br>• Introduction: Supportive image to help clients bring important strengths and qualities to mind or as a general resource to meet important goals<br>• Facilitator example and introduction of the worksheet<br>• Clients completing the worksheet |
| How to take control: compassionate awareness exercise<br>*8–10 min* | Includes<br>• Brief introduction: mention that during the practice clients will be asked to bring to mind a recent mistake<br>• Compassionate awareness exercise (use compassionate awareness prompts) |
| Thinking about the week ahead<br>*2–5 min* | Brief summary of the session<br>Clients identify what they want to do at home |
| Evaluation form | Give participants the sessional evaluation form |

# COMPASSIONATE AWARENESS

Lead through awareness exercise for 8–10 min. Note: The below are prompts which are not intended to be read out like a list but intended to be "dropped into" the practice at appropriate intervals.

- You may want to close your eyes, you don't have to, the reason I suggest it is that it can make it easier to focus on what you have chosen to focus on.
- Take a few moments to become aware of the movement of your breath and the physical sensations in the body.
- When you ready bring your awareness to the sensations of touch and pressure where your body makes contact with the chair.
- Bring a mistake or failure to mind that has been bothering you lately. Something that you may have been criticizing yourself for.
- Whatever this was, trying to get in touch with the feelings you have. What does it make you feel: sad, inadequate, isolated....
- And just begin to get a sense of where you notice these feelings in your body. Allow these feelings to be there.
- If you can, get a sense of any tension or discomfort in the body. We can cause ourselves a lot of suffering by believing we must be perfect, that we can't make mistakes.
- I'm going to repeat some phrases which are designed to help you see that like us all you are an imperfect being, you try your best but nobody is perfect. We all make mistakes, we all fail.
- It is likely that your mind will wander from time to time and if it does, just notice it and gently return your attention to the practice.
- So I'm going to say some phrases and please silently repeat them to yourself if you want to. I'll repeat these phrases a few times.
- May I be safe; may I be kind to myself; may I accept myself as I am.
- Try to get in touch with the feeling behind the words. It can help if you bring to mind the compassionate/nurturing image we were developing to enable you to: draw on the qualities you need and allow yourself to be kind and accepting to yourself. What does the image look like or maybe you just get a sense of the image...
- May I be safe; may I be kind to myself; may I accept myself as I am.
- Giving yourself the same kindness and support as you would be a good friend who was feeling bad.
- Bring to mind any personal strengths or qualities you identified earlier, e.g. I try to be kind
- Keep in mind your strengths; notice if a situation comes to mind in which you can use your strengths to achieve your goals
- And in a few moments, we'll be drawing this practice to a close, so just being aware of this.
- When you are ready, open your eyes and bring your attention back to the room.
- Notice the chair supporting you, and look around you; noticing what you see and hear, now, in this room.

## References

Brunstein, J. C. (1993). Personal goals and subjective well-being: A longitudinal study. *Journal of Personality and Social Psychology, 65*(5), 1061.

Niemiec, R. M. (2013). *VIA character strengths: Research and practice (the first 10 years). Well-being and cultures* (pp. 11–29). New York: Springer.

Sheldon, K. M., & Kasser, T. (1995). Coherence and congruence: Two aspects of personality integration. *Journal of Personality and Social Psychology, 68,* 531–543. Available from https://doi.org/10.1037/0022-3514.68.3.531.

Sheldon, K. M., & Lyubomirsky, S. (2006). How to increase and sustain positive emotion: The effects of expressing gratitude and visualizing best possible selves. *The Journal of Positive Psychology, 1*(2), 73–82. Available from https://doi.org/10.1080/17439760500510676.

Tai, S. J. (2009). Using perceptual control theory and the method of levels to work with people who experience psychosis. *The Cognitive Behaviour Therapist, 2*(03), 227–242. Available from https://doi.org/10.1017/S1754470X09990134.

CHAPTER

# 10

# Session 6 Moving Forward: What Gets Me Stuck, What Helps

## OVERVIEW

As the final session of the Take Control Course (TCC), this sixth session reviews the material covered. It encourages clients to identify elements they found helpful and to consider other resources that they can employ going forward.

The format will be the same for all the chapters in Part B. Slides are number by session and order; for example, the first slide in this session would be 6.1, the second slide 6.2. A condensed session plan is provided after the list of all the session materials. Session worksheets are included on the companion website.

## KEY SESSION FOCUS

The focus of the session is on consolidating what has been learnt and planning for the future. Clients are encouraged to choose elements of the TCC that they want to revisit. Allowing choice in the material covered, and encouraging clients to reflect on what works for them and when, encourages flexible control. Planning for the future uses what perceptual control theory (PCT) describes as the "imagination mode" and the theory behind this is discussed later.

*Transdiagnostic Group Therapy Training and Implementation*
DOI: https://doi.org/10.1016/B978-0-12-813989-9.00010-5

## OVERALL RATIONALE

Throughout the TCC, the material is structured to encourage clients to control in a flexible way. In this context, flexible control refers to the ability to move awareness up and down the control system in order to meet valued goals. Increasing research suggests flexible employment of strategies in accordance with goals is adaptive (Aldao & Nolen-Hoeksema, 2012; Kashdan & Rottenberg, 2010; Kelly, Wood & Mansell, 2012). This session provides the opportunity for clients to identify the understandings and strategies that are enabling them to meet their goals. The key emphasis is on whether such strategies promote achievement of important goals, that is, flexible control, or get in the way and cause conflict.

According to PCT, all action is the control of perception. In a PCT hierarchy, the only point that action meets the environment is at the lowest level loop. All levels above set the desired perceptions for the level below. This is what makes us so flexible under normal conditions. It means that all actions are goal-driven at some level and it is this goal—this perceptual state—that matters. For example, "seeing a friend" is about getting the perception of the friend being with you, however this is achieved. "Reading a book" is about getting the experiences involved in reading that you want, such as excitement, imagery, the feel of the pages. The "action" is potentially variable. For example, someone else could flick the pages, or there could be no pages, such as on an ereader. Higher level goals are key, because they set the reference values for lower level goals, yet higher level goals can only be pursued through their connections to these layers of lower level goals. Awareness of the important perceptual goals to be achieved allows people to adapt their actions and responses to flexibly achieve their goals. So helping people to elaborate on what they expect to experience when they engage in an action can help them to be more adaptive. For example, a client who usually gets help by phoning up their sister, can be asked to encouraged to consider what she is expecting to perceive—a caring voice; time to talk; some reassurance. This frees her up to think of other ways to achieve this.

So we flexibly achieve our goals much of the time, but if there is an unresolved conflict then we will be unable to achieve all of our goals. For example, Laura was experiencing a conflict between "expressing vulnerability to others" and "always appearing emotionally self-contained." She was unable to achieve these goals all of the time and was feeling confused, stressed out, and low. Though attending sessions of the TCC she was able to bring awareness to both goals and a perceptual shift occurred. She realized that both these goals could be helpful depending on the context she is in (e.g., at work or being with a close friend) and accepted that it is OK to be in two minds about this. Based on this realization, she felt much more able to flexibly decide when she was comfortable to express sadness, fear, and mistakes she had made, and when she was not. Moving through this conflict enabled her to control in a flexible way.

## RATIONALE: USING THE "IMAGINATION MODE"

Often controlling experiences involves acting within the world. However, humans also have an internal world of thoughts, imagery, and internal sensations. Within PCT, these internal representations and experiences can be used without direct contact with the environment. This is described as "imagination mode." For example, during the goal-focused exposure exercises within TCC clients are imagining a situation rather than it originating from external sensory input. They are bringing to mind a situation in which important life goals are blocked. From this imagination-based process, clients may experience shifts in their understanding and the resolution of underlying goal conflicts. Often these changes will involve them doing certain things a bit differently.

Another example of the imagination mode is mentally going through a route prior to setting out on a journey. A number of research studies describe the utility of using the imagination in order to plan behavior and evaluate courses of action (Hesslow, 2002; Marks, 1999; Moulton & Kosslyn, 2009). This can enable learning and increased confidence for when the individual is ready to implement the course of action. This planning function of the imagination mode is particularly used in this session to encourage clients to consider any signs that might indicate difficulties, or loss of control, and to consider what they could do if this arose.

## BEFORE THE SESSION

- Set up the room as described in Chapter 4, How to Use This Book, Part A.
- Print out the relevant session handouts (included on the companion website)
- Bring the relevant materials (listed before the condensed session plan on p. 159).

# SESSION SECTIONS

## Overview of Session

Introduce the theme of the session and give a brief overview of what will be covered:

> Different people find different things helpful. You will know best the things that are more and less helpful in managing your anxiety/ problems and enabling you to meet your goals. It can be helpful to consider that you may experience setbacks along the way, for example something very upsetting may happen or your stress may increase. It is normal to experience difficult emotions at times. If you do experience setbacks then this is a time when you can use the techniques you find helpful, although you can certainly use these techniques at other times- in order to maintain control and carry on meeting your goals!

## Continuing to Take Control: Videos

***Materials:***

Slide: "Continuing to take control" (6.2)

*Application and practice.* In both of the videos, Sarah and Sheela describe how they have continued to take control of the problems they were facing. Sarah describes being better able to handle certain situations and feeling that she can control the dread she was experiencing. She says that when she is feeling a bit anxious or facing a challenging situation she finds it helpful to consider how important it is, for example, "is it important what people think?" Sheela describes seeing what she learnt as "good skills for life" that can get her through "hiccups."

*Take home message and linking to previous sessions.* Sarah and Sheela's accounts show that it can be useful to keep using the understandings and approaches learnt, especially during more challenging experiences. Thinking back to "Session 5" these are the resources that we can draw on in order to keep meeting the goals that are most important to us.

## What Have We Covered [See companion website for training video]

***Materials:***

Slide: "What we have covered" (6.3)

Slide: "How to take control" (6.4)

*Take home message.* In this section, we are going to recap the themes and techniques covered within the TCC. Hopefully this will help you to consider which elements you found helpful in meeting your goals. You may also identify that there are some of these elements that you want to continue keeping in mind or acting upon.

Later in the session, we are going to ask you to choose specific elements of the Course that you want to revisit. These could be elements you found helpful, or that you feel that you did not fully "get" before. So it is worth bearing this in mind as we review the elements of the course.

*Application and practice.* Facilitators recap on the themes and techniques covered within the sessions.

The themes were (detailed on slide 6.3 and elaborated upon below):

- Considering how much control we have. Facilitators can refer back to the continuum of control exercise used in Session 1 and 4, saying something like: "throughout the course we considered how much control we have over important areas of our life; for example, we rated our amount of control on a 0–10 scale using the control continuum. We've considered ways in which we can get more control over areas of our life."
- Considering the goals that underlie the problems we are having. Often we experience problems when we are stuck between two different impulses/goals, or two different sides of ourselves. We can feel pushed and pulled, but do not always know exactly what is pulling us.
- Considering whether the strategies we use are helpful short term or long term and looking at whether we prioritize our long-term goals enough. Also noticing that some of the emotions we can see as negative, such as anxiety, can be useful to us (facilitators can refer to the fact that this was explored in the "designing a person from scratch" exercise).
- Considering how we can take control with different people in our lives, which is often not an easy thing to do. We emphasized the importance of keeping in mind the goals that are most important to us when in discussion with other people and looking for goals that are shared. We also talked about clarifying what we want out of the situation, deciding how much we are willing to compromise, saying what we want clearly and assertively.

Techniques, or ways of approaching our experience, that we covered included (detailed on slide 6.4 and elaborated upon below):

- Awareness technique: We used an awareness exercise that involved focusing on sounds and one that involved focusing on bodily sensations.

- Taking control in imagination (Bringing a problematic experiences to mind): We identified a problematic experience that was preventing us from achieving our goals and then brought this experience to mind.
- Upward arrow tool: This can be used to clarify the goals that are most important to us. Often these will be long-term goals.
- PCA (Perceive-Control-Act) problem-solving tool: This can be used to further clarify goals and identify if any conflicted goals are blocking achievement of important goals.
- Supportive image.
- Appreciating our strengths; for example, "Strengths and resources check list". Both the supportive image and the "Strengths and resources check list" can be used to keep in mind our positive qualities and strengths when we are experiencing difficulties. We can use our strengths and resources to take control and meet important goals.

## Thinking About the Future: Video

***Materials:***

Slide: "Thinking about the future" (6.5)
*Application and practice.* Cath talks about noticing that her control has increased since accessing the TCC. She also talks about what her goals are for the future. It is important to her to keep up her current level of control, enjoy life, be happy and be grateful for what she has got. Clients may want to discuss any important goals for the future that struck them while listening to Cath.
*Take home message.* Considering our goals for the future is an important step so we can work out what we need to do achieve these. One of the goals could be keeping up our current level of control or increasing it. In order to achieve either of these goals it can be useful to consider what gives us control.

## Moving Forward: What Gets Me Stuck? What Helps?

***Materials:***

Slide: "Moving forward" (6.6)
Slide: "Moving forward 2" (6.7)
"Moving forward: what gets me stuck? What helps?" worksheet
*Take home message.* In this section we are going to consider what resources, strengths, understandings and activities are helping you

take control. This may include techniques from this course that you are finding helpful. It is important to consider whether these resources, techniques etc. are enabling you to meet your most important goals. We will also consider if there are any situations or events that are/could cause you to feel less in control. This is so that you can consider what could help you through such situations. It is normal that you may experience "setbacks" and difficult emotions at times.

*Application and practice.* Facilitators talk through the questions on the slides (that depict the questions on the "Moving forward: what gets me stuck? What helps?" worksheet). These questions are detailed on slides 6.6.and 6.7 and elaborated upon below.

- *What things are important to me? What type of people do I want in my life? What type of person do I want to be?* Facilitators can suggest clients think back to the upward arrow exercise in Session 4, or other exercises used to clarify goals (e.g., in Session 1).
- *What things are helping me feel in control at the moment?* Facilitators can suggest clients consider the whole course and identify any elements that have been particularly helpful for them. The strengths and resources identified in Session 5 could provide additional ideas.
- *What events/situations cause me to be more vulnerable and feel out of control/stuck?* This could include situations that are currently causing clients difficulties and they may want to consider situations that could be difficult in the future.
- *What are the signs that I'm feeling out of control or stuck? What would I be feeling, thinking and doing?* A range of signs could indicate this. Signs could include levels of stress or anxiety increasing, mood becoming increasingly low, irritability, etc. Facilitators can suggest clients think back to the experiences and behaviors that arose toward the being of their recent difficulties.
- *What can I do to avoid losing control?*
  *What could I do differently? What would work best?*
  *When I'm struggling or feeling bad, what could I do that will help?*

  The understandings and approaches that help clients could be similar to those that they are identified help them maintain control at the moment. But they may identify additional actions, such as going to see their general practitioner (GP) or speaking with a close friend.
- *What strengths, qualities and resources can I draw on if I'm struggling or feeling stuck?*

  Again these maybe similar to the strengths, qualities and resources that are currently helping clients maintain control.

Ask clients to complete the "Moving forward: what gets me stuck? What helps?" worksheet. As ever, while clients are filling in worksheets facilitators offer them support as required; for example, let clients know that they can make eye contact with facilitators or gesture them over if they want to clarify something.

## What Do You Want to Cover?

***Materials:***

Reference slide: "What do you want to cover?" (6.8)
All session worksheets
All session PowerPoint slides

*Application and practice.* Facilitators ask clients what they want to cover in the second half of the session. These could be elements clients found helpful, or felt they did not fully understand before. Usually at least a few clients will have suggestions and facilitators can generally cover three sections (depending how long the earlier material has taken and the length of each component). If there are more components suggested than it is possible to cover, then clients may come to agreement through discussion. Or, if this does not arise fairly quickly, then facilitators can ask clients to vote.

Clients may ask to cover a range of elements. The PCA problem-solving tool and the awareness exercise can commonly be requested, but it varies a lot from group to group. Commonly elements from Session 4, and sometimes Session 5, are requested. Session 4 focuses on control of the environment, including taking control with other people, and it is often the more interpersonal components that clients want to revisit. This seems to reflect the complexity of long-standing interpersonal difficulties for some clients. Again this can be an opportunity to ask clients curious questions regarding a particular interpersonal problem.

Because it is not possible to predict exactly which elements are covered, facilitators should ensure that they feel comfortable explaining all session sections and have the resources available to do so. It can be easier if facilitators cover elements that they have already presented in this course or previous ones; for example, if one facilitator had led most of the awareness exercises or explained the PCA problem-solving tool both times then it makes sense that they would lead these. Ideally both facilitators would lead at least one section. Facilitators should have a brief discussion to agree who is leading what section and what order they will cover the sections.

## Thinking About the Week Ahead

***Materials:***

Reference slide: "Thinking about the week ahead" (6.9)
"Thinking about the week ahead" worksheet
*Take home message.* Different people find different things helpful at different times. In this session you have considered which resources, strengths, understandings, and activities help you manage difficulties and meet your goals. You also identified understandings and techniques that you can take from this course and continue to use.
*Application and practice:* Encourage clients to fill in the "Thinking about the week ahead" worksheet. They may want to identify specific goals for the next few weeks. If they are planning into the future, ways of reminding themselves of what they intended to do could be helpful. For example, they may use post-it notes, or notes in a diary or calendar. They may also want to use photographs or other images to remind them of an important goal/value. If possible, facilitators should give an example of how they use visual images in this way.

# MATERIALS REQUIRED

*Worksheets required:*

All previous session worksheets

*Facilitator prompts required:*

Compassionate awareness
Body awareness prompts
Awareness exercise prompts
Guided exposure in imagination prompts

*Other materials required:*

Post its
Control continuum
Pens
Projector to show PowerPoint slides and videos
Laptop (to use with projector)
Speakers
All previous PowerPoint presentations
Clinical measures

# CONDENSED SESSION PLAN: SESSION 6

| | |
|---|---|
| Measures | Give clients the clinical measures prior to the session |
| Theme/overview *5 min* | Introduce the theme of the session |
| Continuing to take control: Videos *3 min* | Sarah and Sheela describe how they have continued to take control |
| What have we covered *5–10 min* | Facilitators recap the themes and techniques covered within the Take Control Course |
| Thinking about the future: Video *5 min* | Cath talks about her goals for the future |
| Moving forward: what gets me stuck? What helps? *15 min* | Facilitators talk through the "Moving forward: what gets me stuck? What helps?" worksheet and then clients complete |
| | ***SHOULD BE AT LEAST HALFWAY THROUGH*** |
| What do you want to cover? *20–25 min* | Ask clients what they want to cover in the second half of the session and them cover the relevant components |
| Summary *5 min* | Briefly summarize at the end of the group and complete "thinking about the week ahead" worksheet |
| Evaluation form | Give participants the sessional evaluation form. Emphasize the importance of feedback |

## References

Aldao, A., & Nolen-Hoeksema, S. (2012). The influence of context on the implementation of adaptive emotion regulation strategies. *Behaviour Research and Therapy*, *50*(7–8), 493–501. Available from https://doi.org/10.1016/j.brat.2012.04.004.

Hesslow, G. (2002). Conscious thought as simulation of behaviour and perception. *Trends in Cognitive Sciences*, *6*(6), 242–247.

Kashdan, T. B., & Rottenberg, J. (2010). Psychological flexibility as a fundamental aspect of health. *Clinical Psychology Review*, *30*(7), 865–878. Available from https://doi.org/10.1016/j.cpr.2010.03.001.

Kelly, R. E., Wood, A. M., & Mansell, W. (2012). Flexible and tenacious goal pursuit lead to improving well-being in an aging population: a ten-year cohort study. *International Psychogeriatrics*, *1*(1), 1–9. Available from https://doi.org/10.1017/S1041610212001391.

Marks, D. F. (1999). Consciousness, mental imagery and action. *British Journal of Psychology*, *90*(4), 567–585.

Moulton, S. T., & Kosslyn, S. M. (2009). Imagining predictions: mental imagery as mental emulation. *Philosophical Transactions of the Royal Society B: Biological Sciences*, *364*(1521), 1273–1280. Available from https://doi.org/10.1098/rstb.2008.0314.

# PART C

CHAPTER

# 11

# Riding the Waves of Cognitive Behavioral Therapy: Contextualizing the Take Control Course Within Cognitive Behavioral Therapy

This chapter situates the Take Control Course (TCC) in relation to other cognitive behavioral therapy (CBT) interventions. Reading this chapter is likely to enhance the readers understanding of the similarities and differences between TCC and other approaches. We first describe the three "waves" of CBT, and where transdiagnostic approaches fit with these. We then go through examples of forms of CBT that have taken a transdiagnostic approach, describing their conceptual basis and evidence to date. Finally, and importantly, we remind the reader of the distinctive features of perceptual control theory (PCT), and how this entails distinctive features of the TCC, while acknowledging inevitable overlaps. Given both the uniqueness of PCT and its lack of affinity with any particular "wave" of CBT, one could regard the TCC as "riding the waves" of CBT. We hope that by the end of this chapter it will be clear as to the original contribution of the TCC and the features that make it particularly flexible and efficient for many services.

The history of CBT is covered in detail elsewhere (Mansell, 2008a, 2008b; Mansell & Taylor, 2012; Rachman, 1997). Its scientific and philosophical origins are broad and at different phases in its development, CBT has integrated a wide range of earlier work. One of the most critical features to note for the purpose of this manual is that arguably the first ever cognitive therapy—Albert Ellis's rational therapy (Ellis, 1958) – was

*Transdiagnostic Group Therapy Training and Implementation*
DOI: https://doi.org/10.1016/B978-0-12-813989-9.00011-7

not diagnosis driven, but was focused on alleviating psychological distress. It was not until Aaron T. Beck, a psychiatrist, developed and coined "cognitive therapy" that the adherence to a specific diagnosis began—starting with depression in the 1960s and then gradually being tailored to a wide range of different disorder labels throughout the 1980s and 1990s. This period also marks the shift from the first wave (1950s–1970s) when cognitive and behavioral therapies were largely separate, to their fusion as CBT in the 1970s and 1980s, and the emergence of a wide range of "third wave" CBTs from the start of the 1990s. The third wave CBTs tend to focus on a person's relationships with their thoughts rather than addressing biases in thinking directly. However, the conceptual origin of this shift is diverse, and includes eastern philosophy, metacognitive theory, modular theories of cognition and emotion, attachment theory, contextual behaviorism, and self-regulation theory. Given that the third wave CBTs take the stage with the continued practice of first and second wave CBTs, the conceptual basis of CBT is now heterogeneous and lacks a clear consensus (Mansell, 2008a,b).

It is in this confusing context that we developed the TCC, with the hope that its conceptual basis—with only a handful of principles to learn and understand–would provide some clarity. We focused on the consensus that mental health problems are associated with a loss of control, and therefore geared the course around a theory that explains how control works—known as PCT. It is a theory that is grounded in biology and control engineering, which we feel circumvents much of the mixed terminology and assumptions of other theories that have guided CBT to date. We will demonstrate some of the clear contrasts it makes with other theories, and in turn how this can make an important difference to the practice of the TCC.

## THE HISTORY OF THE DEVELOPMENT OF TRANSDIAGNOSTIC COGNITIVE BEHAVIORAL THERAPY

Besides the early origins of rational therapy as a "pre"-diagnostic CBT, the transdiagnostic approach emerged first from second wave CBT. One might question the reason for this development. Since the 1990s, CBT has offered a range of efficacious treatment protocols for targeting specific disorders, as evidenced by a substantial number of randomized controlled trials (RCTs) (for reviews, see Butler, Chapman, Forman & Beck, 2006; Hofmann, Asnaani, Vonk, Sawyer & Fang, 2012). There is now a plurality of disorder-specific protocols within the "CBT family" (Dobson & Beshai, 2013; Mansell, 2008a,b). One key reason for the development of transdiagnostic approaches, cited by Fairburn, Cooper and

Shafran (2003), is that people's diagnosis changes over time. Fairburn et al. (2003) noted that this transition occurred across different eating disorders, leading them to develop a transdiagnostic CBT across the range of eating disorders. Indeed most of the second wave transdiagnostic CBTs have tended to target a specific class of psychological disorder. For example, previous research into transdiagnostic CBT groups has mainly focused on specific populations, such as clients with anxiety disorders (McEvoy, Nathan & Norton, 2009; Norton, Hayes & Springer, 2008), rather than the broad range of problems targeted within TCC.

When the third wave interventions emerged, they typically focused on a specific disorder (Linehan, Armstrong, Suarez, Allmon & Heard, 1991; Segal, Williams & Teasdale, 2002; Wells, 2011). Yet, mindfulness-based therapies and acceptance and commitment therapy (ACT; Hayes, Strosahl, & Wilson, 1999) have embraced the transdiagnostic approach. For example, mindfulness-based stress reduction (MBSR) has been effectively used with clients with a range of physical and psychological difficulties (Baer, 2003; Keng, Smoski & Robins, 2011). ACT has been applied in transdiagnostic samples, including studies comparing ACT to CBT (Newby, McKinnon, Kuyken, Gilbody & Dalgleish, 2015; Rost, Wilson, Buchanan, Hildebrandt & Mutch, 2012; Ruiz, 2012). Other examples of third wave approaches are dialectical behavior therapy (Linehan et al., 1991; Linehan, Bohus, Lynch & Gross, 2007), compassion-focused psychotherapy (Gilbert, 2005; Gilbert & Procter, 2006) and Metacognitive therapy (Wells, 1997, 2011). Again these could potentially be offered on a transdiagnostic basis (Braehler et al., 2013; Goss & Allan, 2010; Neacsiu, Eberle, Kramer, Wiesmann & Linehan, 2014; Nordahl, 2009), but have commonly been delivered in disorder-specific samples.

The key principles of PCT were specified in detail prior to CBT (Powers, 1973; Powers, Clark & Mc Farland, 1960a, b). Therefore, a PCT approach does not align itself with any of the waves, although it does value the contribution of first, second and third wave CBT (Alsawy, Mansell, Carey, McEvoy & Tai, 2014). Therapies and interventions that are informed by PCT take a transdiagnostic approach, because PCT is a broad theory of how psychological distress and psychopathology arises that applies across disorders.

## THE CONCEPTUAL BASIS OF THIRD WAVE TRANSDIAGNOSTIC APPROACHES

This chapter focuses on the theoretical basis of ACT (Hayes et al., 1999) and mindfulness-based interventions. These are provided as examples of influential third wave approaches.

ACT (Hayes et al., 1999) is a psychological intervention based on modern behavioral psychology. It is primarily derived from relational frame theory (RFT; Hayes, Barnes-Holmes & Roche, 2001). RFT proposes that cognition is a specific type of learned behavior, which can influence the effects of other behavioral processes. Events are related on the basis of formal properties (e.g., size, shape) and on the basis of more socially constructed and contextual cues (Hayes, Levin, Plumb-Vilardaga, Villatte & Pistorello, 2013). For example, a range of cues can lead to a child developing the thought that they are inadequate in some way, including responses to academic achievement, bullying, parental separation etc. ACT targets changing the content and impact of cognitive networks through changing their contextual features (Hayes, Luoma, Bond, Masuda & Lillis, 2006). RFT suggests that weak or unhelpful contextual control over language processes themselves results in psychological inflexibility, which in turn leads to psychopathology (Hayes et al., 2006). Psychological inflexibility in this context refers to: "an inability to persist or change behavior in the service of long-term valued ends" (Hayes et al., 2006, p. 6). An example of unhelpful contextual control is when humans predict, evaluate, and avoid "negative" emotions via comparative relations present in language. For example, seeing a thought that "I am unlovable" as objective reality; consequently predicting others will be rejecting or disinterested, and avoiding intimate relationships. Experiential avoidance, such as avoiding the thought of being unlovable and associated feelings, tends to increase the functional importance of the avoided experience (Hayes et al., 2006). For example, for a client who is socially anxious, and avoids anxiety, increasing numbers of situations can be associated with anxiety and therefore avoided. In addition to experiential avoidance, other key processes targeted using ACT are: cognitive fusion, which "refers to verbal dominance over behavioral regulation to the exclusion of other sources of stimulus control" (Hayes et al., 2013, p. 5) and lack of clarity regarding values. See Hayes et al. (2006) for a more detailed account of the theoretical basis of ACT.

In contrast to ACT, a variety of mechanistic and conceptual frameworks have been proposed to understand the utility of mindfulness techniques in clinical contexts. Self-regulatory theoretical frameworks have been cited by a number of authors (e.g., Bishop et al., 2004; Kabat-Zinn, 1982; Tang, Hölzel & Posner, 2015). Self-regulatory theories suggest that cognition and behavior is generally instigated to promote attainment of goals (Carver & Scheier, 1998; Powers, 1973). When an important goal is not, or cannot, be met negative affect and distress occurs. Individuals can try to establish how their goals can be met through rumination (Bishop et al., 2004). Mindfulness-based approaches enable awareness to be directed to distressing or unwanted experiences, without as much discursive thought, thus enabling more directive and less ruminative problem-solving (Baer, 2007; Segal et al., 2002). Mindfulness has been found to increase clarity regarding important goals and promote flexible goal pursuit (Crane, Barnhofer, Hargus, Amarasinghe & Winder, 2010; Crane, Winder, Hargus, Amarasinghe & Barnhofer, 2012). PCT can be described as a self-regulatory theory, so self-regulatory frameworks commonly show some overlap with PCT accounts.

Additional frameworks to explain Mindfulness-based approaches (e.g., Hölzel et al., 2011; Shapiro, Carlson, Astin & Freedman, 2006) include those that provide a broad mechanistic and neurobiological account (Tang et al., 2015; Vago & Silbersweig, 2012). Mindfulness based cognitive therapy (MBCT) is based on an interacting cognitive subsystems framework (Teasdale, Segal & Williams, 1995), which has since been applied to a range of other disorders, such as personality disorders, bipolar disorder, and anorexia (Duff & Kinderman, 2006; Lomax, Barnard & Lam, 2009; Park, Dunn & Barnard, 2011). It is beyond the scope of this chapter to provide a detailed account of interacting cognitive subsystems (see Cowdrey, Lomax, Gregory & Barnard, 2016) and of all the other theoretical accounts of mindfulness.

# EVIDENCE FOR THIRD WAVE AND TRANSDIAGNOSTIC INTERVENTIONS

There are a number of studies investigating whether transdiagnostic and third wave approaches are effective. To illustrate some of this evidence, this chapter will focus on the evidence base for ACT and mindfulness-based interventions delivered in transdiagnostic samples. It will also consider the evidence for the effectiveness of group transdiagnostic "second wave" CBT.

## Mindfulness

Three studies have reported pre-post treatment effects in samples with a range of psychological and physical disorders; all of these studies were of MBSR (Reibel, Greeson, Brainard & Rosenzweig, 2001; Roth & Creaser, 1997; Roth & Robbins, 2004). Psychological diagnostic information was obtained from self-report and medical records, but diagnostic interviews were not conducted. Two of these studies did not have a control group (Reibel et al., 2001; Roth & Creaser, 1997). One had a no treatment control group, but the comparison group was not matched with those receiving treatment and demonstrated differences (e.g., all those in the control group were Hispanic women, whereas the treatment group included both genders and a mix of ethnicities) (Roth & Robbins, 2004). All studies showed significant pre-post improvements on measures of anxiety, self-esteem, and/or depression (Reibel et al., 2001; Roth & Creaser, 1997; Roth & Robbins, 2004). Furthermore, one study included a one-year follow-up and demonstrated significant improvements in depression, and anxiety scores at follow-up (Reibel et al., 2001). Given that the intervention was effective in the absence of diagnostic assessments, having a diagnosis may not be necessary and the intervention may be flexibly adapted to work on client-specified problems. However, the one study that included a no treatment control group only found a trend toward a difference between groups on a measure of quality of life (Roth & Robbins, 2004). One additional study evaluated MBCT in a heterogeneous anxiety and depression sample and found significant improvements in depression, anxiety, stress, and insomnia symptoms (Ree & Craigie, 2007).

Four RCTs are reviewed in more detail elsewhere (Newby et al., 2015). These include three studies evaluating the effects of MBSR with mixed samples (heterogeneous anxiety disorders) (Arch et al., 2013; Kabat-Zinn et al., 1992; Vøllestad, Sivertsen & Nielsen, 2011). One of these samples was followed-up at three-years (Miller, Fletcher & Kabat-Zinn, 1995) and posttreatment reductions in anxiety symptoms were maintained. Further, in another study, MBSR demonstrated greater symptom reductions than wait-list control (Vøllestad et al., 2011) and comparable outcomes to transdiagnostic CBT (Arch et al., 2013).

Overall these studies suggest that mindfulness-based approaches are effective within transdiagnostic samples, but only a limited number of studies included a control group. A greater number of RCTs would be useful in drawing more definite conclusions.

## Acceptance and Commitment Therapy

There have been a number of studies examining ACT in transdiagnostic samples, including studies comparing ACT to CBT. ACT was compared to waiting-list control, and participants accessing ACT demonstrated greater improvements on measures of anxiety and depression (Fledderus, Bohlmeijer, Pieterse & Schreurs, 2012). One RCT, for individuals with cancer, comparing ACT to a CBT-based control condition found that participants accessing ACT demonstrated greater improvements in anxiety, and depression than those accessing the CBT-based control (Rost et al., 2012). However, another RCT comparing ACT to applied relaxation, also in a physical health population, found that depression, and anxiety reduced in both groups (Thorsell et al., 2011). One small rated-blind RCT compared treatment as usual to ACT (plus treatment as usual) for clients with psychosis, and found that reductions in symptoms in those receiving ACT were more marked for depression than anxiety (White et al., 2011). In two studies comparing ACT to traditional CBT, using measures of anxiety and depression, ACT was found generate similar outcomes (Forman, Herbert, Moitra, Yeomans & Geller, 2007), or to be more effective than CBT (Lappalainen et al., 2007). However, 18-month follow-up data for one of these studies found that the CBT group demonstrated greater maintenance of treatment effects for depression and general functioning (Forman et al., 2012).

Overall these studies suggest ACT is probably effective for transdiagnostic samples and that effectiveness is similar to CBT, but there were a number of limits to the studies including small sample sizes, and variance in the interventions offered. Also none of the above studies used diagnostic interviews, and only a limited number used manualized treatment (Newby et al., 2015). One exception is Arch et al. (2012), who compared the efficacy of individual ACT to individual transdiagnostic CBT. There was significant difference between ACT and transdiagnostic CBT at posttreatment. At 12-month follow-up there were lower primary disorder severity ratings for the ACT group (this reached significance in the completer sample only), and CBT clients reported significantly higher quality of life.

Both the ACT and mindfulness-based studies reviewed are part of a wider debate about the use of diagnostic interviews in research into transdiagnostic samples. In clinical practice, diagnostic interviews are not always used, and one of the potential advantages of a transdiagnostic approach is being able to offer an intervention without requiring a diagnostic interview (Morris et al., 2016). Further it can be argued that due to the criticisms of diagnostic classification, and shifts toward more process focused research (e.g., the research domain criteria within the National Institute of Mental Health)(Morris & Cuthbert, 2012), diagnostic ratings should not be considered a key criterion in defining study quality (Atkins et al., 2017). However, it can be counter-argued that without the use of diagnostic interviews it cannot be conclusively demonstrated that an intervention is effective for a range of different disorders or compared to other studies (Öst, 2014, 2017). For pragmatic, and conceptual reasons, a number of studies of transdiagnostic interventions do not include diagnostic interviews (Atkins et al., 2017). But this can lead to criticism regarding the quality of the studies (Öst, 2017).

## Overview of the Evidence for "Second Wave" Transdiagnostic Cognitive Behavioral Therapy

As mentioned previously, transdiagnostic interventions that align themselves with second wave (traditional) CBT commonly target a specific class of psychological disorder. For example, previous research into transdiagnostic CBT groups has mainly focused on specific populations, such as clients with anxiety disorders.

A meta-analysis of transdiagnostic CBT groups for clients with anxiety found a large average effect size ($d=1.29$) (Norton & Philipp, 2008). However, few of the studies reviewed utilized a control group (McEvoy et al., 2009; Norton et al., 2008). A recent meta-analysis combined transdiagnostic and disorder-specific interventions for anxiety disorders to compare effect sizes, utilizing a total of 80 studies (Pearl & Norton, 2017). They found that transdiagnostic interventions were equivalent in effects to disorder-specific interventions, but the transdiagnostic interventions were less affected by comorbidity.

Another meta-analytic review also found reductions in anxiety and depression, although with a smaller effect size than earlier reviews (anxiety $g = 0.85$; depression $g = 0.92$) (Newby et al., 2015). This meta-analysis included a broader range of transdiagnostic interventions than other meta-analyses; including seven mindfulness/acceptance-based interventions (out of 47 studies). The authors found moderate to large overall differences in anxiety and depression severity between transdiagnostic interventions and controls (Newby et al., 2015). Interestingly the review also found that, on average, second wave CBT significantly out-performed third wave treatments in reducing anxiety but not depression. However, there were relatively few studies of third wave therapies, and so results must be interpreted with caution. The authors suggest that it is possible that CBT was more powerful in reducing anxiety overall because exposure-based techniques are included as a core component in these protocols. Exposure has been proposed as a transdiagnostic component of successful psychotherapy (Carey, 2011). However, different therapies focus on exposure to different degrees, and in different ways; for example, exposure to situations evoking fear in imagination and in "real life" (in vivo) is a key component of CBT for phobias, agoraphobia, panic, obsessive-compulsive, and post-traumatic stress disorder (Boswell, Farchione, et al., 2013; Carey, 2011). Although establishing exposure as a causal factor would require empirical validation, it is interesting to note that there can be considerable overlap in the techniques used in different interventions (Arch & Craske, 2008).

The research reviewed finds positive results for the effectiveness of transdiagnostic "second wave" CBT groups. These compare well with both disorder-specific and other transdiagnostic interventions.

## INTERIM SUMMARY

Overall both second wave and third wave CBT group-interventions have positive effectiveness findings (Newby et al., 2015). The degree to which these are offered to clients with a broad range of disorders varies. For example, some interventions are targeted at clients with anxiety disorders (McEvoy et al., 2009; Norton, 2008; Norton & Philipp, 2008). Therefore they still rely on a disorder-based framework. The TCC, on the other hand, has been explicitly designed to target transdiagnostic processes and as such does not require diagnostic assessment to determine whether clients are suitable to access it. This is not to negate the potential utility of more disorder-focused approaches and the value of the process research that underpins them. For example, research into self-reports of control and transdiagnostic processes (e.g., worry, behavioral avoidance) have informed the development of the TCC. But the TCC is focused on client goals and idiosyncratic problems, and it is not targeted at clients within one particular disorder grouping. In this regard, TCC has some similarities with ACT because it is explicitly based on a transdiagnostic theory, it emphasizes client goals or values and it stresses theoretically-driven mediating processes (Atkins et al., 2017).

In spite of its broad transdiagnostic potential, thus far, the TCC has been evaluated in a primary care context. It has also been evaluated as a relatively brief intervention. Until it has been evaluated in other contexts, this is primarily the context in should be offered in. In Part C, Chapter 13, Taking Practice Forward, we discuss potential adaptations to the TCC and ways in which it could be appropriately be offered to other client groups.

## DISTINCTIVENESS AND OVERLAP WITH OTHER TRANSDIAGNOSTIC APPROACHES

### Contrast With Second Wave Transdiagnostic Cognitive Behavioral Therapy

Although transdiagnostic second wave CBT interventions can have some similarities with TCC (e.g., use of exposure techniques), they differ from the TCC in a number of important ways. For example, they focus on traditional CBT techniques (such as cognitive restructuring) and treatment rationale is explained in terms of traditional CBT (such as thoughts, feeling, and behavior cycles) rather than control and goal conflict (Morris et al., 2016). Therefore familiar techniques, such as exposure, are presented and conceptualized differently. According to PCT, exposure is perceptual and not behavioral. This means that people attempt to keep the properties of their experience (e.g., closeness, intensity) within a desired range using dynamic changes in behavior (e.g., movement, using substances) (Brady & Raines, 2009; Carey, 2011). The proposed problem is that people have conflicting perceptual goals; for example, the conflict between avoiding a past memory of a distressing assault, with the need to experience this memory to manage similar situations in the future (Morris, Mansell & McEvoy, 2016). This leads to loss of control as the person oscillates from one goal to the other. Consequently in the TCC exposure is designed to help people hold this perceptual conflict in mind and establish a new organization of goals (reorganization) that allows them to regain overall control (Morris et al., 2016). The way in which the exercise is framed is always in the context of important higher level goals in order to promote awareness of goal-conflict, instead of promoting habituation to anxiety, emotional-processing, or reappraisal of a situation (e.g., Foa et al., 2006). These outcomes may arise, but they are not seen as the reason for exposure. See Morris, Mansell, Amos, and Edge (2016) for additional information on this.

## The Rationale and Practice of Mindfulness in the TCC

The TCC includes mindfulness/awareness techniques. However, awareness techniques used in the TCC are shorter than those delivered in other approaches; for example, MBCT (Fjorback, Arendt, Ørnbøl, Fink & Walach, 2011). This is because the primary reason for using awareness techniques, according to PCT, is to develop present moment awareness that can be brought to bear on conflicted goals (Morris et al., 2016). This enables the reorganization process to happen effectively, because effective reorganization needs to occur at the level of the control system that is setting the conflicted goals. Use of awareness techniques supports clients to sustain attention on problematic experiences indicative of goal conflict (e.g., during the imaginal goal-focused exposure). From a PCT perspective, it is also important that individuals are able to flexibly move awareness through the control hierarchy in order to reduce the likelihood of psychopathology and achieve long-term goals (Watkins, 2011). For example, long-term goals need to be implemented through lower level actions, if awareness is not flexible then it will be difficult to attend to the level within the control system required to meet goals. Emerging research indicates that greater mindfulness is associated with increased clarity regarding important goals and greater flexibility of goal pursuit (Crane et al., 2010; Crane et al., 2012). Enhanced selective and executive attention can be developed through short-term meditation practice and may increase flexibility of awareness; however, it is not clear whether the amount of practice during the TCC would be sufficient (Chiesa, Calati & Serretti, 2011). But TCC participants are provided with support to practice awareness techniques at home if they choose to. Further, even very brief mindfulness conditions have been shown to reduce reactivity to repetitive thoughts (Levin, Hildebrandt, Lillis & Hayes, 2012). See Morris, Mansell, Amos et al. (2016) for additional discussion of this.

## Why Is There Some Overlap Between Therapies?

PCT specifies processes that contribute to psychopathology and psychological change that are relevant to the experience of all psychological disorders. Therefore it would be expected that effective therapies include some similar features. For example, a number of therapeutic approaches include exposure in some form, including ACT, disorder-specific and transdiagnostic second wave CBT and TCC (Barlow, 2004; Carey, 2011; Hayes, 2002; Morris et al., 2016). A comparison between key principles of PCT and familiar psychotherapies is provided in Morris et al. (2016) and an adapted version is reproduced here (see Table 11.1).

Consequently some of the research into transdiagnostic processes is relevant to transdiagnostic CBT, TCC, and mindfulness-based approaches (Baer, 2007; Barlow, 2004; Boswell, Thompson-Hollands, Farchione & Barlow, 2013; Einstein, 2014; Morris et al., 2016). For example, research into rumination is relevant to TCC as repeated and prolonged employment of rumination, which limits attention and disrupts awareness of goal conflict, promotes on-going difficulties (Morris et al., 2016; Watkins, 2008). Another example of process research that is relevant to a range of therapies is the literature on intolerance of uncertainty. Intolerance of uncertainty refers to and has been demonstrated to maintain a number of psychological disorders (Einstein, 2014). While TCC does not directly target intolerance of uncertainty, it recognizes that trying to control the uncontrollable will lead to distress, and that clients often gain from sustaining awareness on the uncertainties surrounding goal conflict (Einstein & Mansell, 2016). Participants are encouraged to reflect on conflicting goals, and to consider what they can and cannot control throughout the TCC, and from this process many participants have reported that they were able to let go of dwelling on concerns that they could not control (Morris, Mansell, Amos et al., 2016).

PCT "surfs the waves" of CBT to provide an integrative approach to understanding psychological distress and recovery. For example, a recent review of fifty studies focused on what makes transdiagnostic processes so problematic that they cause clinically significant distress (Morris & Mansell, in press). Although further research is required in this area, the review indicated that it is inflexibility in the manner in

**TABLE 11.1** Key Principles of PCT and Examples of Similarities/Differences to Familiar Psychotherapies. Based on Table 2 in Morris, Mansell, and McEvoy (2016). The Take Control Course: Conceptual Rationale for the Development of a Transdiagnostic Group for Common Mental Health Problems. *Frontiers in Psychology*

| | Therapy | | | |
|---|---|---|---|---|
| **Principle/Process** | **Take Control Course (Based on PCT)** | **Second Wave CBT**[a] | **Acceptance and Commitment Therapy (Based on RFT)** | **Mindfulness-based Cognitive Therapy (using ICS theoretical perspective)**[a] |
| Control– keeping a perception as close as possible to a desired reference value | Control as fundamental to life; functional process to be restored and refined | Not emphasized, except in some specific models [e.g., Hofmann's (2007) social anxiety model; Fairburn, Shafran and Cooper's (1999) Anorexia model] | Control as problematic (especially regarding internal processes); to be reduced in therapy | Attentional control seen as functional and to be increased |
| Goal conflict- the state when two control systems attempt to control an experience with respect to two (or more) opposing reference values | Higher level goal conflict key source of distress and psychopathology | Not explicitly emphasized, although approach-avoidance conflicts are identified in some models (e.g., Kimbrel, 2008) | Not explicitly targeted, but potentially addressed through acceptance focus | Not emphasized |
| Control hierarchy– internal reference values that are arranged in a hierarchical network | Goals are organized in a complex and many layered hierarchy; eleven layers have been specified | Core beliefs, dysfunctional attitudes, strategies are organized hierarchically. These represent distorted and dysfunctional cognitions rather than goals | Values and specific goals are specified, but hierarchical organization not specified | Nine interacting cognitive subsystems are proposed, some of which are hierarchically arranged; these are specialized for handling a particular type of information |

| | | | | |
|---|---|---|---|---|
| "High-level goals" or "values" identified | Pertinent higher level goals identified through sustained awareness on problems | Not explicitly emphasized. concrete goals for therapy are seen as important, but often not specified in the models used | Values identified through value clarification exercises | Not explicitly emphasized, but can be discussed in regards to relapse prevention |
| Reorganization (and observable indicators)– a trial and error process that makes changes when there is conflict within a control system | Provides a mechanistic account of how change happens, indicated by shifts in perspective/ "insight" moments | Cognitive reappraisal and schematic change could be observable indicators (but not mechanistically specified) | Not specified | Modification of affect-related schema, for example. reducing the likelihood that mild depression will regenerate depressogenic schematic models, could be observable indicator |
| Awareness | An index of the current focus; reorganization occurs at the focus of current awareness | Not emphasized | Targets cognitive defusion and acceptance | Targets attention regulation, acceptance, decentering/ reperceiving (similar to defusion) etc. |

[a]*There is not a universally agreed theoretical basis for mindfulness-based interventions. Interacting cognitive subsystems (ICS) has been proposed as a theoretical account of mindfulness-based cognitive therapy (Teasdale et al., 1995) and is included as it provides a detailed explanation of the ways in which interactions between cognitive and affective processes contribute to psychological distress.*

Note: PCT: Perceptual Control Theory; RFT: Relational Frame Theory; ICS: Interacting Cognitive Subsystems

The purpose of this table is not to provide a comprehensive comparison of therapies. It is focused on PCT-relevant processes; for example, cognitive biases are not included because, while these are fundamental to CBT, they are only significant in a PCT conceptualization to the extent they cause chronic higher level goal conflict. *[Reproduced with permission.]*

which processes are employed that makes them pathologically problematic. A PCT framework was used to explain how and why the evidence pointed to this. The framework presented was that employment of transdiagnostic processes would only become problematic if they impede achievement of another important goal. When such processes are applied rigidly, that is, repetitively and sometimes with limited volitional control, they are more likely to impede goal awareness and attainment (Morris et al., 2016; Teachman, Joormann, Steinman & Gotlib, 2012). Further, an interesting study of the stances (ways people relate) to internal states in a nonclinical sample, investigated whether opposing emotional states (e.g., experiencing emotions verses avoiding emotions; relishing emotions verses eliminating emotions) shared common variance (Hassell & Mansell, 2017). This examined whether the amount of intensity and effort could provide an understanding of why particular stances are problematic and investigated whether such general factors could integrate some of the stances to emotion that are described in different terms and theories. For example, one of the findings of this study was that emotional avoidance was not associated with higher scores of depression, anxiety, and stress, which maybe explained by the PCT understanding that disengagement from unpleasant emotions is only a problem when it interferes with important goals and can be used adaptively (e.g., to concentrate on work). This is interesting given the key importance of experiential avoidance in approaches such as ACT. It could be that research on stances toward emotion could provide very valuable information on what stances will be unhelpful and helpful across therapeutic approaches.

## SUMMARY AND CONCLUSIONS

This chapter has contextualized the TCC within the broader "family" of CBT interventions. It has discussed the similarities and differences between theoretical perspectives and between interventions. It has also described some of the "process research" that applies to a range of different psychological interventions. While some components of TCC could be familiar, it is focused around the concept of control and based on the premise that control is exercised at various levels for a human being to continue living (Morris et al., 2016). Psychological distress is regarded as the manifestation of loss of control, typically caused by prolonged conflict between high-level goals. Therefore, change is promoted by shifting awareness to this conflict and by sufficiently sustaining awareness in order to allow spontaneous changes that resolve the goal conflict. The focus on key mechanisms of control and conflict results in differences between the TCC and other transdiagnostic interventions.

# References


Alsawy, S., Mansell, W., Carey, T. A., Mc Evoy, P., & Tai, S. J. (2014). Science and practice of transdiagnostic CBT: a Perceptual Control Theory (PCT) Approach. *International Journal of Cognitive Therapy, 7*(4), 334–359. Available from https://doi.org/10.1521/ijct.2014.7.4.334.

Arch, J. J., & Craske, M. G. (2008). Acceptance and commitment therapy and cognitive behavioral therapy for anxiety disorders: different treatments, similar mechanisms? *Clinical Psychology: Science and Practice, 15*(4), 263–279.

Arch, J. J., Ayers, C. R., Baker, A., Almklov, E., Dean, D. J., & Craske, M. G. (2013). Randomized clinical trial of adapted mindfulness-based stress reduction versus group cognitive behavioral therapy for heterogeneous anxiety disorders. *Behaviour Research and Therapy, 51*(4), 185–196.

Arch, J. J., Eifert, G. H., Davies, C., Vilardaga, J. C. P., Rose, R. D., & Craske, M. G. (2012). Randomized clinical trial of cognitive behavioral therapy (CBT) versus acceptance and commitment therapy (ACT) for mixed anxiety disorders. *Journal of Consulting and Clinical Psychology, 80*(5), 750.

Atkins, P. W., Ciarrochi, J., Gaudiano, B. A., Bricker, J. B., Donald, J., Rovner, G., … Hayes, S. C. (2017). Departing from the essential features of a high quality systematic review of psychotherapy: A response to Öst (2014) and recommendations for improvement. *Behaviour Research and Therapy.*

Baer, R. A. (2003). Mindfulness training as a clinical intervention: a conceptual and empirical review. *Clinical Psychology: Science and Practice, 10*(2), 125–143.

Baer, R. A. (2007). Mindfulness, assessment, and transdiagnostic processes. *Psychological Inquiry, 18*(4), 238–242.

Barlow, D. H. (2004). *Anxiety and Its Disorders: The Nature and Treatment of Anxiety and Panic.* Guilford press.

Bishop, S. R., Lau, M., Shapiro, S., Carlson, L., Anderson, N. D., Carmody, J., et al. (2004). Mindfulness: a proposed operational definition. *Clinical Psychology: Science and Practice, 11*(3), 230–241.

Boswell, J. F., Farchione, T. J., Sauer-Zavala, S., Murray, H. W., Fortune, M. R., & Barlow, D. H. (2013). Anxiety Sensitivity and Interoceptive Exposure: A Transdiagnostic Construct and Change Strategy. *Behavior Therapy.* Available from https://doi.org/10.1016/j.beth.2013.03.006.

Boswell, J. F., Thompson-Hollands, J., Farchione, T. J., & Barlow, D. H. (2013). Intolerance of Uncertainty: A Common Factor in the Treatment of Emotional Disorders. *Journal of Clinical Psychology, 69*(6), 630–645.

Brady, A., & Raines, D. (2009). Dynamic hierarchies: a control system paradigm for exposure therapy. *The Cognitive Behaviour Therapist, 2*(1), 51–62. Available from https://doi.org/10.1017/S1754470X0800010X.

Braehler, C., Gumley, A., Harper, J., Wallace, S., Norrie, J., & Gilbert, P. (2013). Exploring change processes in compassion focused therapy in psychosis: results of a feasibility randomized controlled trial. *British Journal of Clinical Psychology, 52*(2), 199–214.

Butler, A. C., Chapman, J. E., Forman, E. M., & Beck, A. T. (2006). The empirical status of cognitive-behavioral therapy: a review of meta-analyses. *Clinical Psychology Review, 26*(1), 17–31. Available from https://doi.org/10.1016/j.cpr.2005.07.003.

Carey, T. A. (2011). Exposure and reorganization: the what and how of effective psychotherapy. *Clinical Psychology Review, 31*(2), 236–248. Available from https://doi.org/10.1016/j.cpr.2010.04.004.

Carver, C. S., & Scheier, M. F. (1998). *On the Self-Regulation of Behavior.* Cambridge: Cambridge University Press.

Chiesa, A., Calati, R., & Serretti, A. (2011). Does mindfulness training improve cognitive abilities? A systematic review of neuropsychological findings. *Clinical Psychology Review, 31*(3), 449–464. Available from https://doi.org/10.1016/j.cpr.2010.11.003.

Cowdrey, F., Lomax, C., Gregory, J., & Barnard, P. (2016). Could a unified theory of cognition and emotion further the transdiagnostic perspective? A critical analysis using Interacting Cognitive Subsystems as a case example. *Psychopathology Review.*

Crane, C., Barnhofer, T., Hargus, E., Amarasinghe, M., & Winder, R. (2010). The relationship between dispositional mindfulness and conditional goal setting in depressed patients. *British Journal of Clinical Psychology, 49*(3), 281–290. Available from https://doi.org/10.1348/014466509X455209.

Crane, C., Winder, R., Hargus, E., Amarasinghe, M., & Barnhofer, T. (2012). Effects of mindfulness-based cognitive therapy on specificity of life goals. *Cognitive Therapy and Research, 36*(3), 182–189. Available from https://doi.org/10.1007/s10608-010-9349-4.

Dobson, K., & Beshai, S. (2013). The theory-practice gap in cognitive behavioral therapy: reflections and a modest proposal to bridge the gap. *Behavior Therapy, 44(4)*, 559–567. Available from https://doi.org/10.1016/j.beth.2013.03.002.

Duff, S., & Kinderman, P. (2006). An interacting cognitive subsystems approach to personality disorder. *Clinical Psychology & Psychotherapy, 13*(4), 233–245. Available from https://doi.org/10.1002/cpp.490.

Einstein, D. A. (2014). Extension of the transdiagnostic model to focus on intolerance of uncertainty: a review of the literature and implications for treatment. *Clinical Psychology: Science and Practice, 21*(3), 280–300. Available from https://doi.org/10.1111/cpsp.12077.

Einstein, D. A., & Mansell, W. (2016). The relevance of uncertainty and goal conflict to mental disorders, their prevention and management: a unifying approach. *The Cognitive Behaviour Therapist, 9*, 215–223.

Ellis, A. (1958). Rational psychotherapy. *The Journal of General Psychology, 59*(1), 35–49.

Fairburn, C. G., Cooper, Z., & Shafran, R. (2003). Cognitive behaviour therapy for eating disorders: a "transdiagnostic" theory and treatment. *Behaviour Research and Therapy, 41* (5), 509–528.

Fairburn, C. G., Shafran, R., & Cooper, Z. (1999). A cognitive behavioural theory of anorexia nervosa. *Behaviour Research and Therapy, 37*(1), 1–13.

Fjorback, L., Arendt, M., Ørnbøl, E., Fink, P., & Walach, H. (2011). Mindfulness-based stress reduction and mindfulness-based cognitive therapy–a systematic review of randomized controlled trials. *Acta Psychiatrica Scandinavica, 124*(2), 102–119. Available from https://doi.org/10.1111/j.1600-0447.2011.01704.x.

Fledderus, M., Bohlmeijer, E., Pieterse, M., & Schreurs, K. (2012). Acceptance and commitment therapy as guided self-help for psychological distress and positive mental health: a randomized controlled trial. *Psychological Medicine, 42*(03), 485–495.

Forman, E. M., Herbert, J. D., Moitra, E., Yeomans, P. D., & Geller, P. A. (2007). A randomized controlled effectiveness trial of acceptance and commitment therapy and cognitive therapy for anxiety and depression. *Behavior Modification, 31*(6), 772–799.

Forman, E. M., Shaw, J. A., Goetter, E. M., Herbert, J. D., Park, J. A., & Yuen, E. K. (2012). Long-term follow-up of a randomized controlled trial comparing acceptance and commitment therapy and standard cognitive behavior therapy for anxiety and depression. *Behavior Therapy, 43*(4), 801–811.

Gilbert, P. (2005). *Compassion: Conceptualisations, Research and Use in Psychotherapy.* Routledge.

Gilbert, P., & Procter, S. (2006). Compassionate mind training for people with high shame and self-criticism: overview and pilot study of a group therapy approach. *Clinical Psychology & Psychotherapy, 13*(6), 353–379. Available from https://doi.org/10.1002/cpp.507.

Goss, K., & Allan, S. (2010). Compassion focused therapy for eating disorders. *International Journal of Cognitive Therapy*, *3*(2), 141–158.

Hassell & Mansell (2017). *Stances towards emotion across diverse therapies: What have they all in common? Paper presented at the British Association of Behavioural and Cognitive Psychotherapies Annual Conference*, University of Manchester, Manchester.

Hayes, S. C. (2002). Acceptance, mindfulness, and science. *Clinical Psychology: Science and Practice*, *9*(1), 101–106.

Hayes, S. C., Barnes-Holmes, D., & Roche, B. (2001). *Relational Frame Theory: A Post-Skinnerian Account of Human Language and Cognition*. Springer Science & Business Media.

Hayes, S. C., Levin, M. E., Plumb-Vilardaga, J., Villatte, J. L., & Pistorello, J. (2013). Acceptance and commitment therapy and contextual behavioral science: examining the progress of a distinctive model of behavioral and cognitive therapy. *Behavior Therapy*, *44*(2), 180–198.

Hayes, S. C., Luoma, J. B., Bond, F. W., Masuda, A., & Lillis, J. (2006). Acceptance and commitment therapy: Model, processes and outcomes. *Behaviour Research and Therapy*, *44*(1), 1–25. Available from https://doi.org/10.1016/j.brat.2005.06.006.

Hayes, S. C., Strosahl, K., & Wilson, K. G. (1999). *Acceptance and Commitment Therapy: An experiential Approach to Behavior Change*. New York; London: Guilford Press.

Hofmann, S. G. (2007). Cognitive factors that maintain social anxiety disorder: a comprehensive model and its treatment implications. *Cognitive Behaviour Therapy*, *36*(4), 193–209. Available from https://doi.org/10.1080/16506070701421313.

Hofmann, S. G., Asnaani, A., Vonk, I. J., Sawyer, A. T., & Fang, A. (2012). The efficacy of cognitive behavioral therapy: a review of meta-analyses. *Cognitive Therapy and Research*, *36*(5), 427–440. Available from https://doi.org/10.1007/s10608-012-9476-1.

Hölzel, B. K., Lazar, S. W., Gard, T., Schuman-Olivier, Z., Vago, D. R., & Ott, U. (2011). How does mindfulness meditation work? Proposing mechanisms of action from a conceptual and neural perspective. *Perspectives on Psychological Science*, *6*(6), 537–559. Available from https://doi.org/10.1177/1745691611419671.

Kabat-Zinn, J. (1982). An outpatient program in behavioral medicine for chronic pain patients based on the practice of mindfulness meditation: theoretical considerations and preliminary results. *General Hospital Psychiatry*, *4*(1), 33–47. Available from https://doi.org/10.1016/0163-8343(82)90026-3.

Kabat-Zinn, J., Massion, A. O., Kristeller, J., Peterson, L. G., Fletcher, K. E., Pbert, L., et al. (1992). Effectiveness of a meditation-based stress reduction program in the treatment of anxiety disorders. *The American Journal of Psychiatry*, *149*(7), 936–943.

Keng, S.-L., Smoski, M. J., & Robins, C. J. (2011). Effects of mindfulness on psychological health: areview of empirical studies. *Clinical Psychology Review*, *31*(6), 1041–1056.

Kimbrel, N. A. (2008). A model of the development and maintenance of generalized social phobia. *Clinical Psychology Review*, *28*(4), 592–612.

Lappalainen, R., Lehtonen, T., Skarp, E., Taubert, E., Ojanen, M., & Hayes, S. C. (2007). The impact of CBT and ACT models using psychology trainee therapists: a preliminary controlled effectiveness trial. *Behavior Modification*, *31*(4), 488–511.

Levin, M. E., Hildebrandt, M. J., Lillis, J., & Hayes, S. C. (2012). The impact of treatment components suggested by the psychological flexibility model: a meta-analysis of laboratory-based component studies. *Behavior Therapy*, *43*(4), 741–756. Available from https://doi.org/10.1016/j.beth.2012.05.003.

Linehan, M. M., Armstrong, H. E., Suarez, A., Allmon, D., & Heard, H. L. (1991). Cognitive-behavioral treatment of chronically parasuicidal borderline patients. *Archives of General Psychiatry*, *48*(12), 1060. Available from https://doi.org/10.1001/archpsyc.1991.01810360024003.

Linehan, M. M., Bohus, M., Lynch, T. R., & Gross, J. (2007). *Dialectical behavior therapy for pervasive emotion dysregulation. Handbook of Emotion Regulation* (pp. 581–605).

Lomax, C. L., Barnard, P., & Lam, D. (2009). Cognitive processing in bipolar disorder conceptualized using the interactive cognitive subsystems (ICS) model. *Psychological Medicine*, *39*(05), 773–783. Available from https://doi.org/10.1017/S003329170800425X.

Mansell, W. (2008a). The seven C's of CBT: a consideration of the future challenges for cognitive behaviour therapy. *Behavioural and Cognitive Psychotherapy*, *36*(06), 641–649. Available from https://doi.org/10.1017/S1352465808004700.

Mansell, W. (2008b). What is CBT really and how can we enhance the impact of effective psychotherapies such as CBT? In R. House, & D. Loewenthal (Eds.), *Against and for CBT: Towards a Constructive Dialogue?* Herefordshire, UK: Pccs Books.

Mansell, W., & Taylor, J. (2012). What is CBT and what isn't CBT. In W. Dryden, & R. Branch (Eds.), *The CBT Handbook* (1st ed). London: Sage.

McEvoy, P. M., Nathan, P., & Norton, P. J. (2009). Efficacy of transdiagnostic treatments: a review of published outcome studies and future research directions. *Journal of Cognitive Psychotherapy*, *23*(1), 20–33. Available from https://doi.org/10.1891/0889-8391.23.1.20.

Miller, J. J., Fletcher, K., & Kabat-Zinn, J. (1995). Three-year follow-up and clinical implications of a mindfulness meditation-based stress reduction intervention in the treatment of anxiety disorders. *General Hospital Psychiatry*, *17*(3), 192–200.

Morris, L., Mansell, W., Emsley, R., Bates, R., Comiskey, J., Pistorius, E., et al. (2016). Prospective cohort feasibility study of a transdiagnostic group intervention for common mental health problems: the Take Control Course. *Psychology and Psychotherapy: Theory, Research and Practice*, *89*(2), 163–180. Available from https://doi.org/10.1111/papt.12070.

Morris, L., Mansell, W., & McEvoy, P. (2016). The Take Control Course: conceptual rationale for the development of a transdiagnostic group for common mental health problems. *Frontiers in Psychology*, *7*, 99. Available from https://doi.org/10.3389/fpsyg.2016.00099.

Morris, L. & Mansell, W. (in press). A systematic review of the relationship between rigidity/flexibility and transdiagnostic cognitive and behavioral processes that maintain psychopathology. *Psychopathology Review*.

Morris, L., Mansell, W., Amos, R. & Edge, D. (2016). Experiences of a transdiagnostic group, the Take Control Course, for clients with common mental health problems: a qualitative study. Manuscript submitted for publication.

Morris, S. E., & Cuthbert, B. N. (2012). Research Domain Criteria: cognitive systems, neural circuits, and dimensions of behavior. *Dialogues in Clinical Neuroscience*, *14*(1), 29.

Neacsiu, A. D., Eberle, J. W., Kramer, R., Wiesmann, T., & Linehan, M. M. (2014). Dialectical behavior therapy skills for transdiagnostic emotion dysregulation: a pilot randomized controlled trial. *Behaviour Research and Therapy*, *59*, 40–51.

Newby, J. M., McKinnon, A., Kuyken, W., Gilbody, S., & Dalgleish, T. (2015). Systematic review and meta-analysis of transdiagnostic psychological treatments for anxiety and depressive disorders in adulthood. *Clinical Psychology Review*, *40*, 91–110. Available from https://doi.org/10.1016/j.cpr.2015.06.002.

Nordahl, H. M. (2009). Effectiveness of brief metacognitive therapy versus cognitive-behavioral therapy in a general outpatient setting. *International Journal of Cognitive Therapy*, *2*(2), 152–159.

Norton, P. J. (2008). An open trial of a transdiagnostic cognitive-behavioral group therapy for anxiety disorder. *Behavior Therapy*, *39*(3), 242–250. Available from https://doi.org/10.1016/j.beth.2007.08.002.

Norton, P. J., Hayes, S. A., & Springer, J. R. (2008). Transdiagnostic cognitive-behavioral group therapy for Anxiety:outcome and process. *International Journal of Cognitive Therapy*, *1*(3), 266–279. Available from https://doi.org/10.1521/ijct.2008.1.3.266.

Norton, P. J., & Philipp, L. M. (2008). Transdiagnostic approaches to the treatment of anxiety disorders: a quantitative review. *Psychotherapy, 45*(2), 214–226. Available from https://doi.org/10.1037/0033-3204.45.2.214.

Öst, L.-G. (2014). The efficacy of acceptance and commitment therapy: an updated systematic review and meta-analysis. *Behaviour research and therapy, 61*, 105–121.

Öst, L.-G. (2017). Rebuttal of Atkins et al. (2017) critique of the Öst (2014) meta-analysis of ACT. *Behaviour Research and Therapy, 97*, 273–281.

Park, R. J., Dunn, B. D., & Barnard, P. J. (2011). Schematic models and modes of mind in anorexia nervosa I: a novel process account. *International Journal of Cognitive Therapy, 4*(4), 415–437.

Pearl, S. B., & Norton, P. J. (2017). Transdiagnostic versus diagnosis specific cognitive behavioural therapies for anxiety: a meta-analysis. *Journal of anxiety disorders, 46*, 11–24.

Powers, W. T. (1973). *Behavior: the control of perception*. Chicago, Ill: Aldine.

Powers, W. T., Clark, R., & Mc Farland, R. (1960a). A general feedback theory of human behavior: Part I. *Perceptual and Motor skills, 11*(1), 71–88. Available from https://doi.org/10.2466/pms.1960.11.1.71.

Powers, W. T., Clark, R., & Mc Farland, R. (1960b). A general feedback theory of human behavior: Part II. *Perceptual and Motor Skills, 11*(3), 309–323. Available from https://doi.org/10.2466/pms.1960.11.3.309.

Rachman, S. (1997). The evolution of cognitive behaviour therapy. In D. M. Clark, & C. G. Fairburn (Eds.), *Science and Practice of Cognitive Behaviour Therapy* (pp. 3–26). New York, NY, US: Oxford University Press.

Ree, M. J., & Craigie, M. A. (2007). Outcomes following mindfulness-based cognitive therapy in a heterogeneous sample of adult outpatients. *Behaviour Change, 24*(02), 70–86.

Reibel, D. K., Greeson, J. M., Brainard, G. C., & Rosenzweig, S. (2001). Mindfulness-based stress reduction and health-related quality of life in a heterogeneous patient population. *General Hospital Psychiatry, 23*(4), 183–192.

Rost, A. D., Wilson, K., Buchanan, E., Hildebrandt, M. J., & Mutch, D. (2012). Improving psychological adjustment among late-stage ovarian cancer patients: examining the role of avoidance in treatment. *Cognitive and Behavioral Practice, 19*(4), 508–517.

Roth, B., & Creaser, T. (1997). Mindfulness meditation-based stress reduction: experience with a bilingual inner-city program. *The Nurse Practitioner, 22*(3), 150–178.

Roth, B., & Robbins, D. (2004). Mindfulness-based stress reduction and health-related quality of life: findings from a bilingual inner-city patient population. *Psychosomatic Medicine, 66*(1), 113–123.

Ruiz, F. J. (2012). Acceptance and commitment therapy versus traditional cognitive behavioral therapy: a systematic review and meta-analysis of current empirical evidence. *International Journal of Psychology and Psychological Therapy, 12*(3), 333–358.

Segal, Z. V., Williams, J. M. G., & Teasdale, J. D. (2002). *Mindfulness-based cognitive therapy for depression: a new approach to preventing relapse*. New York; London: Guilford Press.

Shapiro, S. L., Carlson, L. E., Astin, J. A., & Freedman, B. (2006). Mechanisms of mindfulness. *Journal of Clinical Psychology, 62*(3), 373–386. Available from https://doi.org/10.1002/jclp.20237.

Tang, Y.-Y., Hölzel, B. K., & Posner, M. I. (2015). The neuroscience of mindfulness meditation. *Nature Reviews Neuroscience*.

Teachman, B. A., Joormann, J., Steinman, S. A., & Gotlib, I. H. (2012). Automaticity in anxiety disorders and major depressive disorder. *Clinical Psychology Review, 32*(6), 575–603. Available from https://doi.org/10.1016/j.cpr.2012.06.004.

Teasdale, J. D., Segal, Z., & Williams, J. M. G. (1995). How does cognitive therapy prevent depressive relapse and why should attentional control (mindfulness) training help? *Behaviour Research and therapy, 33*(1), 25–39. Available from https://doi.org/10.1016/0005-7967(94)E0011-7.

Thorsell, J., Finnes, A., Dahl, J., Lundgren, T., Gybrant, M., Gordh, T., et al. (2011). A comparative study of 2 manual-based self-help interventions, acceptance and commitment therapy and applied relaxation, for persons with chronic pain. *The Clinical Journal of Pain*, 27(8), 716–723.

Vago, D. R., & Silbersweig, D. A. (2012). Self-awareness, self-regulation, and self-transcendence (S-ART): a framework for understanding the neurobiological mechanisms of mindfulness. *Frontiers in Human Neuroscience*, 6, 296.

Vøllestad, J., Sivertsen, B., & Nielsen, G. H. (2011). Mindfulness-based stress reduction for patients with anxiety disorders: evaluation in a randomized controlled trial. *Behaviour Research and Therapy*, *49*(4), 281–288.

Watkins, E. (2008). Constructive and unconstructive repetitive thought. *Psychological Bulletin*, *134*, 163. Available from https://doi.org/10.1037/0033-2909.134.2.163.

Watkins, E. (2011). Dysregulation in level of goal and action identification across psychological disorders. *Clinical Psychology Review*, *31*(2), 260–278. Available from https://doi.org/10.1016/j.cpr.2010.05.004.

Wells, A. (1997). *Cognitive therapy of anxiety disorders*. Chichester, UK: J. Wiley & sons.

Wells, A. (2011). *Metacognitive therapy for anxiety and depression*. London, UK: Guilford press.

White, R., Gumley, A., McTaggart, J., Rattrie, L., McConville, D., Cleare, S., et al. (2011). A feasibility study of acceptance and commitment therapy for emotional dysfunction following psychosis. *Behaviour Research and Therapy*, *49*(12), 901–907.

CHAPTER

# 12

# Embracing the Diversity Within the Course: Revisiting Theory and Practice to Address Clients' Personal Concerns

The aim of this chapter is to revisit the principles of perceptual control theory (PCT) to show in more detail how to help the Take Control Course (TCC) run smoothly. In particular, we address how to work with clients' questions and how to help them when they get stuck.

Let us revisit the aims of the TCC. Ultimately, it is a way to provide a transdiagnostic intervention informed by PCT to a large group of clients, and without a need for disclosure. This fits a clear niche. Some people prefer a "course" to the one-to-one interaction of individual therapy, and there are potential benefits both in terms of client experience and efficiency of delivery. For example, a number of clients who were interviewed about their experience of attending TCC described appreciating the informality and the permission to be flexible in responding to problems provided by a group approach. Some clients specifically stated that they preferred this to a one-to-one approach, as they felt more able to go at their own pace (Morris, Mansell, Amos & Edge, 2016). However, method of levels (MOL), the individual therapy informed by PCT, does work much more directly on the core mechanism of change than the TCC. The experiential exercises in the TCC are just one part of each session. We believe that these are an essential component because they allow the clients to put their understanding into practice by holding a problem situation in mind for long enough for reorganization to make a difference. However, we also accept that this is more challenging in a group context because it is not supported by a therapist's regular questioning.

*Transdiagnostic Group Therapy Training and Implementation*
DOI: https://doi.org/10.1016/B978-0-12-813989-9.00012-9

In contrast, MOL is designed to help the client regain overall control of important aspects of their lives by focusing the client's awareness on their current experience throughout each session to allow time for reorganization to make trial-and-error adjustments. Regular, brief, present-moment focused questions help to sustain this process. The MOL therapist does not need to describe the principles of the theory to the client because their standpoint from which the therapist asks each question takes these into account.

The MOL therapist has two goals—to ask about a current problem and to notice disruptions. The way that a therapist follows the goals is up to the therapist in the moment—there are no specific techniques. However, a general principle is that the therapist needs to only say what they need to say to achieve one of these goals. Saying anything else, and taking valuable attention away from the client's own perspective—is not MOL. Tim Carey puts this neatly with the title of his book, MOL: How to Do Psychotherapy Without Getting in the Way (Carey, 2006).

The disruptions that occur spontaneously when a person talks about a problem they are experiencing are extremely diverse and momentary. They may include changing topic, pausing, moving eyes, emphasizing certain words, gestures, smiles, and other expressions of affect. Disruptions are regarded as an observable sign of a background thought. A background thought is any perception (thought, image, sensation, memory, impulse) at the edge of a client's awareness that they have not put into words. When the MOL therapist notices the disruption, they give the client the opportunity to put that thought into words—if they want to. Asking about disruptions helps the client to focus on the present moment, broaden their description of a problem, sustain awareness on difficult experiences, and notice conflicts. Ultimately however, asking about disruptions helps a client to "go up levels"—to notice the overarching goal that is driving the conflict and undermining their control. According to PCT, it is from this higher level perspective, above the goal conflict, that change through reorganization can work on resolving it. Because reorganization is a trial-and-error process and it takes time to stumble upon a helpful solution or perspective, the MOL therapist continues to help the client keep their awareness there for as long as the client wants to. In sum, MOL is centered around the individual client, helps them to put their unique experiences into words, and heightens focus on current experience.

There is a clear contrast between TCC and MOL. Clients in the TCC cannot be expect to follow the same pace of change. They may follow it at very different paces from one another, and a proportion of them can get stuck with the course at various points because of their individual difficulties. Yet, as you have read so far, the facilitators in the TCC are critical not just in explaining and managing the exercises, but also in answering clients' questions, and in relating to the clients on the course in a manner that is consistent with the principles of the course. Very often therefore, we find that we use a MOL style of questioning with TCC clients to help them clarify a problem and to notice background thoughts about it that they may, or may not, be willing to disclose. At other times, clients may be better served by direct answers or explanations. We will endeavor in this chapter to illustrate how to be sensitive to these different requirements.

Specifically, we have found it helpful to consider three factors that characterize clients' "stuckness." They follow naturally from the PCT account, and they are directly addressed by a MOL approach. These are chronic lack of control, limited awareness of higher level goals, and the uniqueness of each client's problems.

## CHRONIC LACK OF CONTROL

According to PCT, psychological distress is loss of control. Our clients have experienced a prolonged inability to control important aspects of their lives. This often entails that, to compensate, other people have a greater effect on them than they would like. For example, one client felt that her work life was prescribed by her boss and she was very anxious about offering any suggestions for how her role could be different, despite desperately wanting to make significant changes. Having a chronic lack of control also often entails great efforts to try to re-establish control, but in ways that backfire or lead to further difficulties. People may report doing this in angry outbursts, through trying to avoid stressful situations, through suppression emotions, and through alcohol and medication. Chronic loss of control over what is important in one's life can also breed a sense of hopelessness about the chances of regaining control in the future. In practice, this can involve disengagement from friends, disengagement from work, and disillusionment with society.

### How Lack of Control Affects the Take Control Course

Clients attending the TCC sometimes get stuck on the exercises because of their chronic experience of low levels of control. For example, when asked to rate the continuum of control (Session 1), some report, "I find it hard to think of anything I can control" and "It is hard to think how anything would ever look different." When considering the nature of their problems (Session 1, Chapter 5), they may simply feel that everything in their life is out of control, and that other people determine their difficulties. They may also struggle to think of any aspects of their lives, the want to take control of when completing the Perceive-Compare-Act cycles (Session 2, Chapter 6). Taking one further example, they may be so used to their bodily reactions being "triggered" by other people and situations, that they may be convinced that these feelings are completely out of their control.

## Our Approach

It is important to remember that we are fully expecting our clients to not feel in control of their lives, and therefore to struggle to think of what they can control, or change. Their experience of losing control of their lives and not finding a way to fix it is most probably why they are coming to the course. It is valid to feel this way. In fact, compared to a traditional cognitive behavioral therapy (CBT) approach that puts the focus on people's biases in thinking and interpretation of their experiences, PCT states simply that people perceive they have little control over their lives because they do not have control over their lives. There is no need to think that they are distorted in their thinking and just "believe" that they don't have control. As a facilitator, reminding yourself of this view may help to limit your own frustrations if clients struggle with the tasks. It should allow you to talk to the clients in the group such that you honestly and effortlessly validate their experiences and their difficulties.

We also find it helpful as facilitators to remember that the PCT model proposes that conflict is at the root of loss of control. Both sides of conflict can be highly active and involve effort—but if they are pitched directly against one another, they will not move that person an inch. For example, one client put huge efforts into trying to be perfect by checking and rechecking every appliance in her house, only to put even more effort into berating herself for appearing "obsessive" and "crazy" to other people because of the results of her checking. When she eventually began to feel normal for a while this felt empty and unsatisfying, and she then returned to striving for perfection through checking. It can feel all the more frustrating for our clients because we are often told that effort or willpower is what people need to recover from their mental health problems. PCT states clearly that it is not.

Because PCT states that conflict is the most common, and yet often subtle, driver for loss of control, the TCC does not try to help people regain control by encouraging them to put in more effort into controlling, by having more will power, setting up incentives, or by pushing themselves in some way. We are not even asking patients to "try" to change. Any effort they might make in the course goes into keeping their awareness on thoughts and feelings relating to their difficulties for longer so that new perspectives on them emerge naturally. So, while it is very rewarding for facilitators to see clients make changes, we are not expecting changes from everyone, and we are not trying to push people to change. We are not trying to get our clients to "do" anything more than they are doing at the moment. By remembering this principle, it makes it much easier as a facilitator to not set high expectations, to validate lack of progress, and to embrace people's diversity in their rates of progress. You can authentically claim that people should not feel ashamed of "not trying hard enough" by pointing to this paradox of conflict—trying harder makes it worse when in conflict. If clients are willing, you can use their own personal examples to illustrate this occurring.

When our clients tell us that other people are in control of their lives, this must also be taken at face value rather than as a distortion of some kind. It is both a cause and consequence of their own loss of control. Our clients may well have a history of being controlled by parents or other caregivers during childhood, and right now, family, friends and colleagues may be trying to control their lives because they cannot manage to exert control themselves. But again it comes down to conflict. It is only a problem for other people to control your life if they do not manage to get you what you want, or there is something about how they do it that is not what you want. The goal of the course is not for people to take back control of everything in their life so that they no longer depend on other people, or are influenced by them. The aim is to help clients become more aware of what they want to control in their lives and to explore these desires and needs, and any conflicts between them, to be in a position to experience them to the level they want. There may be many aspects of their lives they are less bothered about controlling for themselves. One clear example here is people who have a religious belief, or a belief in fate or God's will. If the person currently sees no difficulty in delegating this aspect of their lives to a force outside themselves, then that should be taken at face value. Of course, they may change this perspective over time, but that should be taken at face value too. Taking these points on board, facilitators should expect some clients to state that parts of their lives are controlled by others. The natural question is to ask what aspects of being controlled by others is a problem. This may reveal the sources of conflict through an MOL style of questioning.

In the course, when we introduce the idea of conflict, it also frees up the facilitators from another, related issue regarding control. Very often clients initially approach the course with a need for information and answers to their questions. When the facilitator points to conflict being at the heart of a problem, it can take a while to get used to. People are very used to being told that certain activities are helpful—exercise, expressing emotions, thinking positive—and certain activities are unhelpful—worry, avoidance, thinking negatively. The TCC facilitator never carves up what a person does in this way. Everything someone does has a reason for doing it, and a potential problem—a conflict with an important goal—that it entails. We find that clients come to see the benefits of this stance as the course progresses, and more widely, it appears to be associated with a greater tolerance of uncertainty generally. That's not to say there are not direct answers for many questions—for example, about how the fight-or-flight system works, or about how control works—it is just that there are no general answers as to whether a thinking style or behavior is either "good" or "bad" (Morris & Mansell, in press).

**Example**

Michael was experiencing a whole range of difficulties, including anxiety, irritability, and depression. He was quite open about his sense of hopelessness and he would struggle to think of anything in his life that he could control.

Michael: "I can't fill in these notes with an example. I just can't think of anything I can control in my life."
Facilitator: "Thanks for mentioning this, Michael. It may be something that a few of you are thinking?" [nods from three people in the group]. "This happens quite often in the first session because the kind of difficulties you are coming to the course to work on are about not being in control. It doesn't matter if you only write down things that you feel you have no control over at all. And we are not trying to get you to overcome these problems right now. The point of the task is just to see if, given a bit of thought, you can notice some things that you have at least a little bit of control over. Michael, do you want me to try to help you identify something you have control over?"
Michael: "Yes, I am fine with that."
Facilitator: "OK, thanks Michael, just tell me if you want to stop at any point. If you think about your daily routine, is there anything that you control?"
Michael: "I don't really have a routine. I just do things when they come up. Sorry!"
Facilitator: "It's not a problem if you can't think of anything right now. Was there anything about coming here today that you were in control of?"
Michael: "I came because my GP said it might help."
Facilitator: "Uh, huh. And today when you made it here, who controlled that?"
Michael: "My wife had to remind me and drive me here."
Facilitator: "OK, so I can see how a lot of the things you do are being influenced by other people. Did you make the choice to come here in the end, or not do you think?"

Michael: "Yes, I guess so." [smiles]
Facilitator: "Was there something else you were going to say?"
Michael: "Yes" [smiles again] "I said to my wife – 'I've got to try something and it's all about taking control and I need that!' – it was odd really."
Facilitator: "What do you mean by odd?"
Michael: "Well I was embarrassed about coming here but I wanted to get help, so I made it here."
Facilitator: "And how does it feel right now?"
Michael: "It feels OK. It is a bit embarrassing talking in front of other people, but its not as difficult as I had thought."
Facilitator: "So is coming here today something you could give a number to – having some control over?"
Michael: "I'd give it a 3 or 4 I think."
Facilitator: "Was that OK asking you these questions?"
Michael: "Yes, it was helpful actually."
Facilitator: "Just say – and this applies to anyone here – I might be curious and ask questions if you have a question for me, but you actually don't have to answer it. I'll check in with you, but do say if you can. It can be helpful to explore people's problems in the course, but it's absolutely not necessary. Michael, do you mind if I mention your dilemma about coming here again?"
Michael: "Go ahead, if you think it will help people here."
Facilitator: "I just wanted to point out that it seemed that you have good reasons to not come to this course – to not feel embarrassed – and good reasons to come to the course – to get help. That's when things get difficult and we can get stuck – when we are pulled two ways like this. It's the conflict. And we will be covering it in more detail later on in the course. Thanks again Michael. Anything you want to add?"
Michael: "No, I'll let everyone get on with the task now!"
Facilitator: "Great, but please anyone who does have a question as we go along, it can be really helpful like Michael's, so please do just ask."

In this vignette, the facilitator is working from the principles of PCT. The first explanation reminds people that often the kind of difficulties that bring people to the course are ones they do not have control of. And so, it is hard to think of things one has control over. This may feel "normalizing" for the clients on the course, but that is not the intention—it is just a fact that emerges from the theory. The facilitator then gets consent from the client to ask further to help him find something he controls. The facilitator chooses to embark on a line of questioning starting with a concrete experience—his daily routine. The client does not immediately think of something. At this point the facilitator could have asked more detailed questions—"What was the first thing you did this morning?"—for example. However, she decides to try an avenue with potentially a greater chance of success—coming to the session. Again, this does not immediately reveal anything the client feels that he controls. The facilitator keeps asking around the topic, making it clear she is listening at the same time. She then notices a disruption—the smile—which she chooses to ask about, but in a way that does not draw excessive attention to it—"Was there something else you were about to say?" The aim of asking about disruptions is to give the client an opportunity to put into words a background thought. This can often reveal a goal conflict, and in this case it did. The facilitator helps the client expand on it with further curious questioning and then asks permission to share it as an example to the group. Throughout there is the reminder that just because this client is sharing a personal experience, it is not necessary or required, and everyone can choose whether or not to talk. She also makes it clear that questions are helpful. This particularly seemed to be the case on this occasion, because it showed that some level of control can be identified with a particular experience, it led to an illustration of the way to ask questions that raise awareness, and it provided an example of conflict.

## LIMITED AWARENESS OF HIGHER LEVEL GOALS

PCT describes at least eleven levels of perception, each of which have desired states (goals), and this number is almost certainly an underestimate. We cannot be aware of all of these levels at any one time. Indeed, we probably spend most of our time with awareness at one level, and maybe two or three at most during our most reflective moments! None of us are aware of our deeper motives as we engage in everyday activities, and rarely do we second guess our own "hidden agenda" when we talk to others, making requests, asking questions, giving suggestions, etc. But this is as it should be. Bill Powers once said "There's no point in reorganizing your religion when working out how to tie your shoe laces!" There is a reason that awareness is not on our higher level goals most of the time—it would be highly distracting, unnecessary, inefficient, and may lead to more problems than it tried to fix! It's also worth remembering that if the clients on the TCC course could already clearly see the problems in their life from the perspective of their higher level goals and the conflicts they might involve, they probably would not need the course. If the TCC clients were at ease with thinking about their conflicts, feeling their associated emotions, and they felt comfortable expressing this, then they would be well along the way to addressing their difficulties. The point of the course is to help people shift from a position at which the root of their difficulties is outside their awareness, to one at which they are able and willing to keep their attention on these experiences. This road to widened awareness is likely to be paved with many obstacles, and these will inevitable arise on the course.

## How It Affects the Take Control Course

Many elements of the course are direct attempts to help people "go up levels" with respect to their problems. Within Method of Levels (MOL), this is achieved through well-paced, brief questions that help draw out people's background thoughts. Within the TCC, it is attempted though a more direct method that is not immediately tailored to the individual. The most obvious examples of this are the Perceive-Compare-Act problem-solving tool and the upward arrow technique. While some people seem to grasp these methods straight away, others will draw a blank the first time they try it. Clients have said to us, "I can't think of anything to fill in here," "I don't have any reasons for this problem - it is just a problem and I don't know why it's there."

It is also the case that clients on the course may hold certain values that impact on their experience of the course without being directly aware of this. For example, clients often come to the course to take responsibility for some of their difficulties but at the same time feel wary of the effects of blaming themselves. They may ask questions that indirectly relate to these goals, such as "What is it that causes someone to worry?", "I don't have any control over my worry so I would rather not write it down." These can sometimes stump facilitators because the clients are not engaging in the task. It can also sometimes lead to discussions that are not within the remit of the course; in this example, it might lead to speculations regarding the "causes" of worry—genetics, learning it from other people, reinforcement. While there is nothing intrinsically wrong with doing this, it does take away the time that the facilitator can be imparting the principles of the course. So, whenever possible we encourage facilitators not to divert from the main aims of the session, or from its principles.

## Our Approach

The starting point for our approach to dealing with lack of awareness of higher level goals is to remember that it is to be expected. More than that, it is very adaptive most of the time not to allow our attention to be drawn to our longer term goals and deeper values.

The upward arrow task can be easily adapted to help clients access at least some higher level goals. First, for any problem the client identifies, the aim is to ask people why it is important for them to address their problems—not to necessarily think about why they have their problems in the first place. For many habitual activities—worry, smoking, and avoiding eye contact, for example—it will be hard for people to begin to think about the possible functions of these activities. However, they may be more readily able to describe why they want to address the problem—namely, what goals the activity interferes with, and therefore what could they achieve if they were to address them. Second, through varying one's questioning in simple ways, it can make a difference. For example one can ask "what difference does it make when you do this?", "what makes it important?', "what would happen if you didn't do it?". Each of these questions may tap into a higher level goal. Third, we find that some sustained questioning about the activity can free the client up, just as an MOL therapist would do: "How much do you worry?", "Are there any times you don't worry?", "What is going on when you start worrying?", "And when you stop?", "How much worry is OK for you?". By being curious about the activity in this way, a clue to a higher order goal may emerge. Alternatively, a disruption is likely to occur as the client is talking. Asking about disruptions needs to be done sensitively bearing in mind the public context. For example, rather than pointing out a nonverbal sign explicitly, one might ask, "Is there something you were about to add there?", "As you are telling me, what else are you thinking?", "I'm just wondering whether your smile means you've noticed something?". One advantage of running the TCC in pairs is that while clients are carrying out a task, both facilitators can go around the room and check in with people to answer questions and stay with a client to use MOL if they are stuck. At other times, it may be necessary to do this in front of the group, and therefore to check with clients that they are comfortable and have the option to have their queries addressed separately if necessary.

We find that it is always helpful to have in mind that what a client says is only a snippet—an "output"—to achieve another goal. The purpose of a question is not necessarily what it appears to be. So, it is appropriate to say, "If you don't mind me asking, why are you asking?" or "Do you mind telling me a bit more about what you have in mind before I answer?". Some people are very willing and able to shed light on their motives when given this opportunity, and it helps to prevent the client and facilitator talking at "cross-purposes." They can then both concentrate on clarifying the real issue, rather than necessarily how it appeared from the question. Remember, from the principles of the course, your job is not to solve people's problems. It is to offer them a different way of understanding their problems—as problems with control, undermined by conflict, that requires sustained attention and consideration before reorganization tumbles upon a possible solution. Therefore, by not trying to answer a question immediately, and by trying to clarify what the client is saying through your curious questions, you are modeling the means of solving problems that we think can work for our clients.

**Example**

The following vignette describes an exchange between a facilitator and a client who cannot at first complete the upward arrow task.

Client: "I've put down that I want to stop being so perfectionist, but I don't know why. I just am - it's my personality."
Facilitator: "That's OK. Actually, what we are trying to get you to do here is to tell us how things might be different if you had more control over your perfectionism."
Client: "It's just the way I am. I've always been like it though."
Facilitator: "So, if you carried on being as perfectionist as you are now, what would happen?"
Client: "I think I would drive everyone away! I do need to keep a lid on it sometimes."
Facilitator: "Ah, so if you were less perfectionist, you'd be less likely to drive people away?"
Client: "Yes, if I could."
Facilitator: "How near do you want people to stay?"
Client: "Closer than they are now" [looks upset] "I want to be closer to my family. If I was less of a perfectionist, I think I'd be easier to live with. But I've tried."
Facilitator: "You want to be less perfectionist to be easier to live with, but it just doesn't seem possible?"
Client: "Yes, that's it. I'd be able to manage work better too. But I always feel I need to get everything exactly right. I have to check I've done my work correctly though. I can't let it go."
Facilitator: "So it seems like you've actually got two reasons to be less perfectionist - to be closer to your family and to manage work better. What would that do for you?"
Client: "It seems impossible right now, but it would make me feel better about myself."
Facilitator: "So you have something to fill in now?"
Client: "I guess so - in another universe!"
Facilitator: "If its OK with you, that doesn't matter - it just about telling us your ideals."
Client: "Thank you."
Facilitator: "Incidentally, what do you think the perfectionism does for you?"

Client: "Makes me feel like I am doing the right thing - being a good person - feeling better about myself!" [laughs]
Facilitator: "What are you noticing there?"
Client: "I want to stop being a perfectionist to feel better about myself and I want to be a perfectionist to feel better about myself. Is that what you call conflict?"
Facilitator: "It's part of it yes. I am getting the impression this might be a something to keep focus on as you do the rest of the session today?"
Client: "It's important to me, so I will."
Facilitator: "Great. Is that OK for now?"
Client: "That's made it a lot easier. I am getting to see the point of all these questions and boxes."

This exchange was precipitated by the client's lack of awareness of their higher level goals, coupled with a strong impression that they had no control over the problem—the perfectionism. This may indeed by the case, but the facilitator indicated that the client could still do the task hypothetically. Doing so, actually freed her up to not only describe the higher level goals in conflict, but to see that both were being driven by one overarching goal—to feel good about herself. From this perspective, whether or not to be perfectionist seemed paradoxical—the conflict seemed self-evident. To get to this point the facilitator used questions to help the client talk about the problem of perfectionism in more depth, as well as noticing disruptions. Such sudden shifts of awareness are not always obvious during the TCC itself, but they do illustrate the ideal path that clients can take when they persist, with the help of facilitators.

## THE UNIQUENESS OF EACH CLIENT'S PROBLEMS

Every client's problems are unique. This is exactly why the TCC is transdiagnostic. It does not attempt to generalize problems into categories that fit a certain diagnosis. PCT reminds us that the pattern of experiences and constellation of goals that each of us holds is unique to each of us. We can never literally see the world through another person's eyes; experience is unique; and each person's range of desired experiences is unique too. Yet, simultaneously, the principles that we use to organize our experiences are the same for everyone. We control them by remembering our desired states for these experiences and act to keep them there. We balance these desired states—goals—with one another and organize them in levels to keep our concepts of ourselves, and our world as we would like them. We resolve conflict between our goals, and we need to allow our minds to shift, and stay with the source of these conflicts to resolve them. So, when you grasp PCT, you give up convincing yourself that you can impart your interpretation of a client's own problems to them. But you gain by appreciating that all problems have the same basic structure, irrespective of their personal content.

## How It Affects the Take Control Course

People are used to being given advice, and to being categorized along with others. A mental health diagnosis has the potential benefit of making it feel that you are like other people with the same diagnosis, and not alone. But it does not work so well when the other people with the same diagnosis are self-evidently different. The TCC is deliberately designed not to fall into this trap. But this does not prevent clients from expecting that they should find similarities between the nature of their problems and the nature of other peoples. When they do not, it creates distance, and possible a lack of investment in the course.

In MOL therapy, personal uniqueness is embraced. The therapist does not expect to understand a client's difficulties, and does not need to understand the difficulties to provide the most effective help possible—to shift and sustain awareness on a problem. The principles of control, levels, conflict, and reorganization covered in the TCC are universal and are obviously not in themselves even a sign of mental health problems. However, inevitably, the cases used in examples and videos each describe a certain type of problem, and when clients choose to share their problems in the course, differences are evident. Some of these differences may themselves be a source of distress—"The lady on the video is no way as severe as me", "I feel as though the course isn't for me because no one else here has had severe depression." It can lead to conflicts between members of a course if they try to give advice that the person receiving it feels would not apply to them. For some people, their sense of difference may make it hard for them to think of any examples for the exercises because their experiences seem so different from the ones used.

## Our Approach

We have found that understanding PCT helps us to genuinely embrace every client's unique problems. This helps us to not assume that one client's way of managing could or should work for someone else. It helps us to be genuinely curious, open about our limitations, and to not take an expert role on how to solve other people's problems. It stops us from attempting to make spontaneous formulations or explanations on the spot. This is not to say that our role is passive or purely reflective. The aim as a facilitator is to try hard to help the person focus on a problem if they choose to do this openly in a session, and to draw out the common principles shared by everyone in the room—we all control; our problems have many levels; we all experience conflict; and we all need time and space to reorganize.

By accepting this as a facilitator, it actually holds a huge advantage. You do not have to completely understand what clients are telling you. You just need to say or do something that helps the person understand themselves and their own social world in a deeper or more detailed way. The facilitator's job is to help clients to see the similarities at the right level—the principles of control, conflict and reorganization—and also in basic shared biology (e.g., fight-or-flight)—rather than trying to see the similarities in other ways, such as the severity of symptoms, and the degree of impact on relationships.

Religious concepts and cultural beliefs can be an important part of an individual's hierarchy—that is, guiding important goals. Within MOL therapy, clients can clarify and explore these experiences and beliefs to the degree they want to do so. This opportunity can also be provided within the course either during a session or within a brief meeting outside it. A PCT framework does not in any way oppose specific religious frameworks, or specify cultural or ethnic norms. It can be used creatively to explore and clarify the meaning and implications of the individual's religious and cultural framework. For example, even when the facilitator might have specific views on a subject from their own cultural experience, they would not impose these on the client. One client was experiencing a lot of distress regarding feeling unhappy in an arranged marriage. Although she felt unhappy, she felt that she would not be a "Good Muslim" if she took these feelings further or ended the relationship. Both a Muslim or non-Muslim facilitator could disagree with this (depending on a number of factors); however, the techniques within a PCT approach are geared around enabling that individual to work through the conflict in light of their own beliefs and context. This individual was able to become more aware of the conflict and felt better in herself, but also decided to stay in her marriage even though she still did not feel happy within it (her goal of being a "Good Muslim" and the implications of this for life after death were more important to her).

**Example**

One client in the TCC was quite troubled by the fact that his difficulties were very different from those in the video examples, and from what he could discern form what other clients had described. He decided therefore to write a summary of the history of his problems for the facilitators to read. It appears that he wanted them to understand him, and to appreciate that he was different. This vignette describes how the facilitators worked with this challenge, for which they had agreed to talk to him privately for 10 minutes before the session.

Facilitator: "We've both had a chance to read the letter you gave us last week. You've clearly had a tough time with everything that's been going on in the last few years. Do you feel that it has helped to write it all down for us?"
Client: "I just wanted you to know what I've been through, and why I might not be getting as much out of the course as everyone else."
Facilitator: "OK, so how did you feel after you'd written it all down?"
Client: "Ermm. Do you mean how did I feel when I'd typed it and printed it out for you?"
Facilitator: "Yes, and while you were typing it out?"
Client: "It felt like a bit of relief really."
Facilitator: "Relief from what?"
Client: "I was thinking you'd understand now, why I find it so hard to change."
Facilitator: "OK. You know it doesn't matter to us how quickly people change, and we really don't know whether this course will be enough at all for you, or for anyone. The course is just one opportunity people have to make a difference. We do want to try our best to get the basic messages across though. Is that working for you yet?"
Client: "I don't get it yet. No one seems to have the same kind of problems as me."
Facilitator: "That's right. Everyone's problems are very different. I couldn't imagine to be in the position you were in that you told us about in the letter. How are you coping at the moment?"
Client: "I'm managing. It's not the life I want."
Facilitator: "I guess one of the ideas we are trying to get across in the course is that it is possible to imagine the life you want - how you want things to be - a piece at a time."
Client: "That's not enough though is it? And how can you help when my problems are so different?"
Facilitator: "Is there something that you want to be different today?"
Client: "I want to sort out this mess that I am in, what I told you about in the letter."
Facilitator: "That makes sense. What bit could you sort out first?"
Client: "I don't know. I need to stop thinking so much about it and get on with my life I guess."
Facilitator: "Which bit of your life is more important right now?"

Client: "You've got me thinking now. Which bit? If I am being honest, it's my relationship with my son. Not because that will sort it all out. Just because I just have so much regret. But I can't forgive him at the same time."
Facilitator: "So there is a lot of mess to sort out that is very different from other people's problems here on the course, but you've started on something there?"
Client: "You got me thinking about that, yes."
Facilitator: "It sounds as though you want a better relationship with your son but you also can't forgive him."
Client: "That's just one of my problems, yes."
Facilitator: "Would you see it as an example of a conflict?"
Client: "Yes, it is that yes."
Facilitator: "Everyone's conflicts are different. Yours is particular to you."
Client: "I can see that other people might have conflicts about people close to them like me."
Facilitator: "Would it sit with you better if your problems were different from everyone else?"
Client: "I can see what you are saying. I am different, but it's still a conflict. That's one of the messages of the course, is that right?"
Facilitator: "Yes, that's it. As its time, are you OK to leave it there and we can join everyone?"
Client: "It's been good to talk about it, thanks."

The facilitator chose to strike a balance between describing the aims of the course, and using a MOL approach in her questions. She wanted to first ask what writing the letter in itself had achieved, in case the client had found that expressing himself in writing had made a difference. However, it did seem to be that the idea of being understood that was his goal. Therefore, the facilitator decided to validate this goal, and ask more about his difficulties to continue on this theme. She tried to focus on a problem going on right now, as one would do in MOL, which actually entailed detecting a conflict. Tentatively, she was able to show that this was a commonality with others that could be used in the course.

## SUMMARY

Following a full explanation of the TCC in the first part of the manual, we introduced this chapter to help new facilitators to think in more depth about how to manage challenges that arise in the course. We saw that most of the challenges are to be expected. First, the very reason that clients may be keen to attend the course is because they experience a chronic lack of control over important aspects of their lives, yet this can make it hard to even begin to talk about the notion of regaining control. Second, it is the norm for our higher level goals to be outside awareness; the course is designed to help people shift their awareness to them, but for many clients that can be experienced as a challenge. Third, the group approach of the TCC requires facilitators to be flexible and curious to respond to client's individual problems. Throughout the chapter, we showed that using a MOL approach with individual clients can help to address each of these challenges, while illustrating the common principles thought to be shared by all long-term mental health problems. Ultimately however, we advocate using client feedback regularly to check in with how well these kinds of challenges are being addressed and to adapt your approach accordingly (Table 12.1). In the spirit of reorganization, if you don't succeed, try something different!

**TABLE 12.1** The Themes of This Chapter Are Recapped in the Summary Table

| Nature of client's concern | PCT explanation | Examples of how it could be approached |
|---|---|---|
| Experiencing very little control | Psychological distress is a chronic loss of control over an important aspect of one's life. However it is not loss of control over *every* aspect of one's life | Remember that the aim of the course is not to try harder to control but to be better at thinking about what we want to control, what we can control to some degree, and where conflicts are undermining control. Method of Levels questions can be used to do this |
| Being unable to access higher level goals | It is not an everyday requirement to be aware of one's higher level goals; in fact in can be distracting. Psychological distress is maintained by an inability or unwillingness to attend to higher level goals, and so may explain why the course is being attended | Remember how normal it is not to have this awareness of higher-level goals, and to use Method of Levels questioning to raise awareness of higher level goals and conflict |
| Focusing on the uniqueness of one's own problems | Everyone has unique perceptions of themselves and the world, and a unique constellation of goals for these experiences. The course focuses on the unifying principles for these, not shared content | PCT explains exactly *why* people have unique problems. Through Method of Levels questioning, clients can share their unique situation as well as begin to notice the common principles behind the nature of psychological distress for everyone |

## References

Carey, T. A. (2006). *The method of levels: How to do psychotherapy without getting in the way.* Hayward, CA: Living Control Systems Publishing.

Morris, L., Mansell, W., Amos, R., & Edge, D. (2016). Experiences of a transdiagnostic group, the Take Control Course, for clients with common mental health problems: a qualitative study. Manuscript Submitted for Publications.

Morris, L., & Mansell, W. (in press). A systematic review of the relationship between rigidity/flexibility and transdiagnostic cognitive and behavioral processes that maintain psychopathology. Psychopathology Review.

CHAPTER

# 13

# Taking Practice Forward

In this final chapter, we outline how the Take Control Course (TCC) can be developed in different services. We discuss how clinicians can develop their skills in delivering TCC, and how the TCC can be adapted for different service contexts.

## DEVELOPING YOUR PRACTICE

We suggest training to deliver the TCC through reading of the manual, repeated practice, and evaluation by yourself and others. If at least one facilitator has previous training and experience in delivering groups then this is beneficial. Although aspects of the TCC can be practiced through delivering them to colleagues, it is useful to have some prior experience in working with groups where possible. If neither of the facilitators have previous experience working with groups, then self-monitoring and supervision is even more important than usual (see next section "evaluating your practice").

A number of aspects of the TCC can be practiced before delivering the course to clients. For example, it is helpful to practice interactive exercises—even if this is just with your co-facilitator—to establish who is doing what and the sequence of steps involved in the exercise.

Another useful way of preparing is practicing curious questioning. This questioning style can be used for any problem that a person is willing to discuss. The problem does not need to be a mental health one; it can be something more general like maintaining a work life balance. It is not helpful to "role play" curious questioning, as it requires accessing real thoughts and behaviors. There are a number of methods to practice curious questioning:

- Working in pairs and each person takes it in turn to talk about a real situation or problem.

*Transdiagnostic Group Therapy Training and Implementation*
DOI: https://doi.org/10.1016/B978-0-12-813989-9.00013-0

- As above, except a third person observes the session. This helps provide another source for feedback. The individuals in the trio rotate roles.
- One person is a client and two or more clinicians take it in turn to ask curious questions.

There is an established psychological intervention based on this curious questioning style, method of levels (MOL). For more details on curious questioning and MOL the interested reader is directed toward: Mansell, Carey, and Tai (2013).

General information and resources regarding applying perceptual control theory (PCT) to mental health problems can be found at: http://www.pctweb.org/psy/mental.html, and the MOL website is http://www.methodoflevels.com.au.

### Further Training

As well as specific training in the TCC, training in MOL can also be highly beneficial in helping obtain a clearer understanding of PCT and what a PCT-based therapy looks like in practice. Training sessions are regularly offered at national and international conferences; for example, the annual BABCP (British Association of Behavioral and Cognitive Psychotherapies) conference.

## EVALUATING YOUR PRACTICE

We recommend that all clinicians access supervision while delivering the TCC. As with any psychological intervention, complex clinical issues can arise. However, due to the considerable resources that are provided to help facilitate the TCC (e.g., worksheets, presentations, this manual!) questions about the content of the sessions are less frequent than in totally open-ended forms of therapy.

It is also recommended that clinicians evaluate their own practice through the adherence scale provided in Appendix D (and on the companion website). This can identify areas to discuss in formal supervision, and can be a useful basis for peer debrief and supervision with their co-facilitator. Someone (who is sufficiently familiar with the TCC) coming into a session can rate the session and provide feedback. Again this feedback can be used to identify supervision and training needs.

## ADAPTING THE TAKE CONTROL COURSE

TCC was designed to be offered within primary care contexts. Given that PCT is a transdiagnostic theory, it is suggested that TCC could be adapted for other client groups. For example, currently an adapted version of the TCC is being developed for adolescents.

The extent to which adaptations are required will depend on how different the service context is. For example, based on experience within the research and clinical group if the TCC is offered to clients with long-term physical health conditions, who primarily want support with anxiety, depression and related problems, then the TCC can require little (if any) adaption.

However, where clients have more dissimilar psychological problems to those found in primary care, greater adaptions will be required. For example, if offering the TCC to clients with addictive disorders a number of changes could be made. One change could be to the focus of the session on "what blocks our control" (Session 2) and this could focus on control of urges to partake in substances, for example, by prioritizing other goals and increased awareness, rather than on repetitive thinking (Fujita, 2011; Thomsen, 2015; Webb, Sniehotta, and Michie, 2010). Although PCT is a transdiagnostic theory, this does not mean that there cannot be differences in the likely content of goal conflicts within different presenting problems. However, because such presenting problems would still be underpinned by self-regulation difficulties resulting from goal conflict, much of the intervention content used to address these conflicts would be similar. As aforementioned, if you were interested in providing the course beyond primary care then we would encourage you to contact us and we can work together on adapting it.

## Delivery Format

One future adaptation to the TCC is offering it within a rolling format. This would entail having TCCs running back to back and offering clients the option of reviewing sessions by accessing the course again. Although this promotes optimum client choice and control, service set-up can make this difficult to implement. For example, many services use electronic systems that are premised on the fact that clients come and access a discrete episode of therapy. However, with increasing use of self-referral in some services, as well as the common experience that certain clients access multiple therapies (e.g., Richards and Suckling, 2009), this option could become more feasible in the future. Such an approach would work particularly well in large groups, but in smaller groups (e.g., <15) this could be experienced as disjointed as closer relationships are likely have developed within the group.

An inspirational example of using larger group formats to make psychological therapies widely accessible is that of the STEPs program in Glasgow (White, 2010). This research group also provides evidence that psychological change can be achieved in primary care through large group courses (White, 1998; White and Keenan, 1990; White, Keenan, and Brooks, 1992). The format of their courses suggests that such groups should not rely on participant disclosure and discussion. Similarly the TCC relies upon experiential exercises, videos, worksheets, and facilitator presentations; consequently it has the potential to be offered to large groups.

## References

Fujita, K. (2011). On conceptualizing self-control as more than the effortful inhibition of impulses. *Personality and Social Psychology Review*, *15*(4), 352–366. Available from https://doi.org/10.1177/1088868311411165.

Richards, D. A., & Suckling, R. (2009). Improving access to psychological therapies: phase IV prospective cohort study. *British Journal of Clinical Psychology*, *48*(4), 377–396. Available from https://doi.org/10.1348/014466509X405178.

Thomsen, K. R. (2015). Measuring anhedonia: impaired ability to pursue, experience, and learn about reward. *Frontiers in Psychology*, (6), 1409.

Webb, T. L., Sniehotta, F. F., & Michie, S. (2010). Using theories of behavior change to inform interventions for addictive behaviors. *Addiction*, *105*(11), 1879–1892. Available from https://doi.org/10.1111/j.1360-0443.2010.03028.x.

White, J. (1998). "Stress control" large group therapy for generalized anxiety disorder: two year follow-up. *Behavioral and Cognitive Psychotherapy*, *26*(3), 237–245.

White, J. (2010). The STEPS model: a high volume, multi-level, multi-purpose approach to address common mental health problems. In J. Bennett-Levy, D. Richards, P. Farrand, H. Christensen, K. Griffiths, D. Kavanagh, & C. Williams (Eds.), *Oxford Guide to Low Intensity CBT Interventions. United States*, New York: Oxford University Press.

White, J., & Keenan, M. (1990). Stress control: a pilot study of large group therapy for generalized anxiety disorder. *Behavioral Psychotherapy*, *18*(02), 143–146. Available from https://doi.org/10.1017/S0141347300018267.

White, J., Keenan, M., & Brooks, N. (1992). Stress control: a controlled comparative investigation of large group therapy for generalized anxiety disorder. *Behavioral Psychotherapy*, *20*(2), 97–113. Available from https://doi.org/10.1017/S014134730001689X.

## Useful Websites

http://www.methodoflevels.com.au
http://www.pctweb.org/psy/mental.html

## Further Reading

Morris, L., Mansell, W., & Mc Evoy, P. (2016). The Take Control Course: conceptual rationale for the development of a transdiagnostic group for common mental health problems. *Frontiers in Psychology*. Available from https://doi.org/10.3389/fpsyg.2016.00099.

### ***Therapy manual for PCT in individual therapy***

Mansell, W., Carey, T. A., & Tai, S. J. (2012). *A transdiagnostic approach to CBT using method of levels therapy: distinctive features*. New York: Routledge.

APPENDIX

# A

# Accessibility, Clarity, and Ease of Use of the Take Control Course Manual: A Qualitative Study

## INTRODUCTION

The Take Control Course (TCC) manual was developed to aid delivery of the Take Control Course, and to contain both the theoretical underpinnings and information on the practical delivery of the course. As part of ensuring the manual was accessible and easy to understand a qualitative study was conducted. Feedback and potential suggestions to aid usability were sought. Five semi-structured interviews took place with Psychological Wellbeing Practitioners or Trainee Psychological Wellbeing Practitioners (see recruitment and participants section for more details). The questions were pre-determined by Dr. Lydia Morris (LM) and Tanya Wallwork (TW). Findings were then analyzed, discussed and adaptations were made.

## METHOD

### Recruitment and Participants

The manual was offered to eight Psychological Wellbeing Practitioners employed by Six Degrees Social Enterprise (Salford, Greater Manchester, UK). Of these eight practitioners, six were qualified Psychological Wellbeing Practitioners and two were trainee

Psychological Wellbeing Practitioners. All clinicians were degree educated and had completed, or were in the process of completing, 1-year further training to deliver low-intensity treatments[1]. The manual was not offered to members of the nonclinical or management teams. Also excluded were any practitioners that had attended the one-day Take Control training workshop delivered by LM.

All eight practitioners were instructed to read the manual as a whole and given a four-month period to complete this. Of the eight practitioners invited to read the manual, five attended the interviews. Three did not attend the interview due to either absence or leaving Six Degrees Social Enterprise. Of the five interviewed two were male (both qualified practitioners) and three were female (two qualified and one trainee practitioner). The five practitioners who attended interviews had received a variety of trainings; for example, they possessed varied degrees of understanding of low-intensity Cognitive Behavioral Therapy (CBT), a minority had received brief training on mindfulness or Perceptual Control Theory (PCT)-informed interventions (i.e., method of levels).

All practitioners that attended the interviews answered the same eight questions that had been pre-determined by TW and LM. These questions covered areas such as whether the manual was understood, whether explanations were credible and clear, whether anything could be added to enhance understanding or clarity.

## Interviews

TW conducted all of the semi-structured interviews with the five practitioners. Each interview was conducted face-to-face and was digitally recorded. Length of interviews was between 6 minutes and 14 minutes long; practitioners were not given a set time frame for interviewing. Each interview was stored on a password protected Dictaphone carried by TW. All participants gave informed consent and provided information regarding the evaluation of the manual.

## Data Analysis

TW and LM agreed, prior to interviews, that the data would be analyzed using Thematic Analysis. The analysis followed all six phases of the Braun and Clarke's (2006) approach; familiarizing yourself with your data, generating initial codes, searching for themes, reviewing themes, defining and naming themes, producing the report.

[1]This training focuses on low-intensity CBT with a particular emphasis on treating anxiety and depressive disorders.

## RESULTS

After all stages of coding and searches for themes were completed, four themes were identified: "Good overall understanding (with sub-themes: last chapter and PCT)," "Part A too long," "Additional resources," and "Confidence in implementation." See Fig. A.1 for initial thematic map.

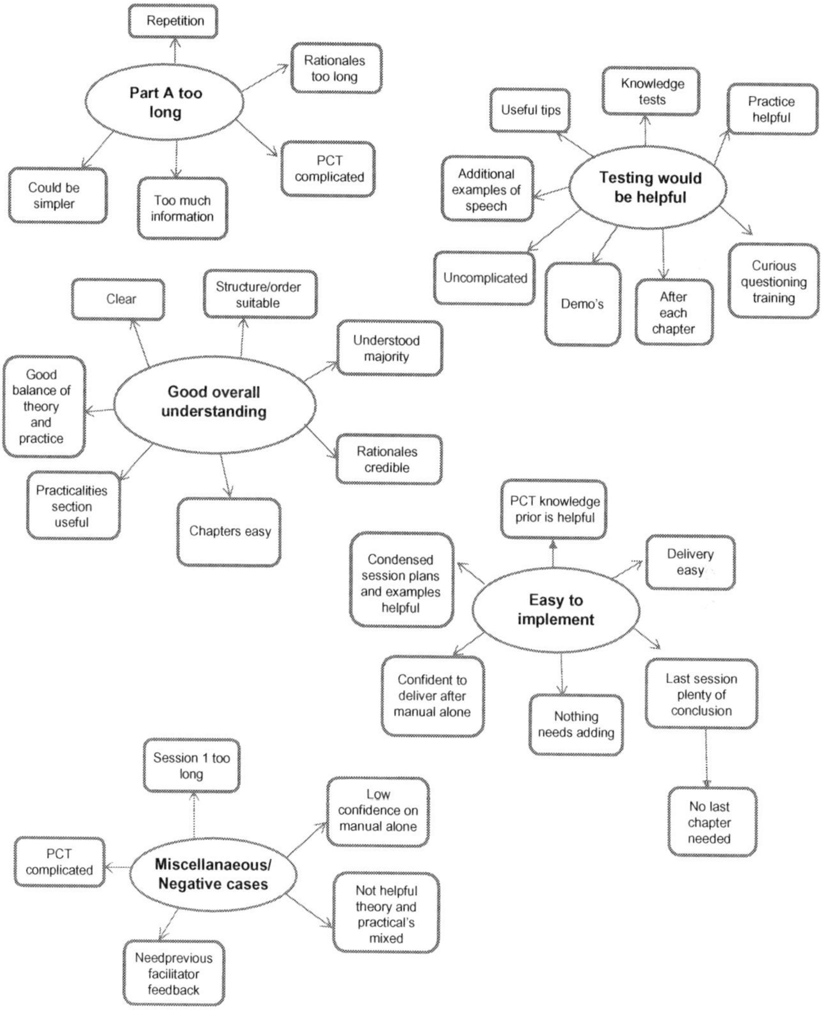


FIGURE A.1 Initial thematic map, showing five main themes.

## Good Overall Understanding

Nearly all the participants stated that they had good overall understanding of the manual as a whole *"I think it was clear and concise all the way through. I think it had theory and practical parts to it that made sense and were very easy to understand and take in (Audio 4)."*

The majority of the participants commented that the structure was suitable *"I would say the structure was quite good (Audio 4)"* and the rationales credible *"I found that the rationales were ok (Audio 5)."*

There was only one participant who noted that having the theory and practical sections mixed was not helpful *"It felt like the theory was interspersed in the practical stuff and I would have liked all the theory together and the practical stuff all together (Audio 5)."*

**Last Chapter.** All five participants agreed a last chapter was not required in the manual *"No I don't think a last chapter was necessary, I think it was pretty straight forward (Audio 2)."*

**PCT.** PCT aspects of the manual were mentioned during the interviews. One participant noted that the PCT components were too complicated: *"but I found the PCT theory it's quite long-winded and some of the explanations were a bit confusing (Audio 2)."* Another suggested that prior PCT knowledge/awareness was helpful in better understanding the manual *"I think the fact that I have got experience in areas that are maybe similar or linked to some of the rationale's that are in there, gives me an advantage that I could understand quite a lot of it (Audio 4),"* with a further comment that it could be simpler for non-PCT readers *"but I think that maybe someone that didn't quite of much of a background may need a little bit more of an explanation on some of the rationales (Audio 4)."*

However, overall the comments regarding PCT were minimal with many of the other comments suggesting participants had a good overall understanding of the manual, including the PCT aspects of it.

## Part A Too Long

The majority of participants suggested Part A was too long. Three out of five of the participants stated Part A contained too much information *"it was a bit wordy in some of the information in part A, I felt was a bit unnecessary (Audio 1)"* with two participants noting that the rationales, while credible, were too long *"I thought the rationale could be a bit more brief and I didn't think it was that necessary in each session to have such a long rationale (Audio 2)."* Two participants commented that some of the content was repetitive *"I did think some of the stuff was a bit repetitive (Audio 5)."*

## Additional Resources

Nearly all participants commented that additional resources would be helpful. Participants gave suggestions for the types of additions they felt that they would benefit from and the frequency of these.

Three out of five of the participants felt that some form of testing of their knowledge would be helpful *"I thought it would* (be useful to have something to test knowledge), *but given that some of the sessions are quite information intensive probably better to keep it something light maybe sort of pub quiz type thing (Audio 1)"; "A little quiz then to check your knowledge then that would be good as well" (Audio 2).* In addition, one participant suggested testing after each chapter: *"I think maybe like a few questions about theories or concepts at the end of each chapter might be useful in terms of testing what you have just read rather than just sort of hoping you had remembered (Audio 4),"* with another commenting that practice alone was needed *"No I don't think so, just need to get on and do it really (Audio 5)."*

Similarly, three out of five participants felt that visual demos would enhance their understanding of sections of the manual *"Maybe like links to video clips just to see it in practice would be good (Audio 2)."*

Two participants felt that curious questioning training would be beneficial: *"the opportunity for some training around asking curious questions might be useful (Audio 1)."* One participant suggested that examples of this in written speech bubble form would be useful *"examples of what you could actually almost learn off by heart would be really helpful, if that was in a box or if it was in italics (Audio 5)."*

## Confidence in Implementation

Confidence in delivering the course after reading the manual was positive.

Two out of five participants felt that delivery would be easy *"I think pretty confident yeah (Audio 4)."* A further two suggested high confidence in their ability to deliver the course from solely reading the manual *"Out of 10 I would say 8, I thought it was pretty clearly explained and there was a lot of detail and it answered most of the questions I would have expected (Audio 1)."*

Two participants suggested that session guides (more detailed versions of the condensed session plans that were being piloted during the project) or examples would be helpful in aiding confidence *"I like the condensed session plan for each chapter that's brilliant (Audio 2)."*

However, one participant noted low confidence in implementation of the course from solely reading the manual *"I personally don't think I could just read this manual and then go deliver a course I think I would need some training or maybe shadow someone else delivering the course first (Audio 3)."*

## DISCUSSION

Overall, the study provided useful insights into the usability and understanding of the manual as a whole. This was apparent in the consistent rating of good overall understanding and confidence in implementation across the interviews. It also highlighted areas that could be improved. A consistent finding was that participants suggested that additional resources would aid usability. This led to suggestions of useful improvements, many of the suggestions were recurrent across the interviews, including a test your knowledge quiz, and video demonstrations. Both of these additions and improvements were implemented.

It worth noting that there are some limitations to this study. Firstly, all participants worked for the same company, which delivers psychological interventions to the same client group (predominately clients with mild to moderate depression and anxiety). While it was helpful to test the manual with a range of therapeutic experiences (from trainee clinicians with very limited therapy experience to clinicians with more than five years' experience), it would be helpful to repeat this study within a different service in order to ascertain whether understanding and usability were still consistently high within other service settings. This would also enable the improvements to the manual following this study (e.g., training videos, quizzes, clarification of structure, edits for concision etc.) to be evaluated. Furthermore, if this study were to be repeated, it would also be helpful to have a second researcher coding to reduce potential bias.

There was one area that drastic changes were not made in response to feedback; this was the suggestion by some participants that the amount of material regarding theory-practice links should be reduced (particularly that Part A should be considerably cut down). Substantial changes were not made in this area as the manual is explicitly theory driven and such elements are integral to the overall objectives of the manual. However, it was made more explicit that the manual is theory driven and some simplifications were made.

Overall, the study was useful and has led to a number of changes and additions to the manual, including but not limited to, extended session sheets, live video demonstrations, trouble shooting challenges with the use of curious questioning, and more detailed condensed session guides.

APPENDIX

# B

# Overview of All the Sessions

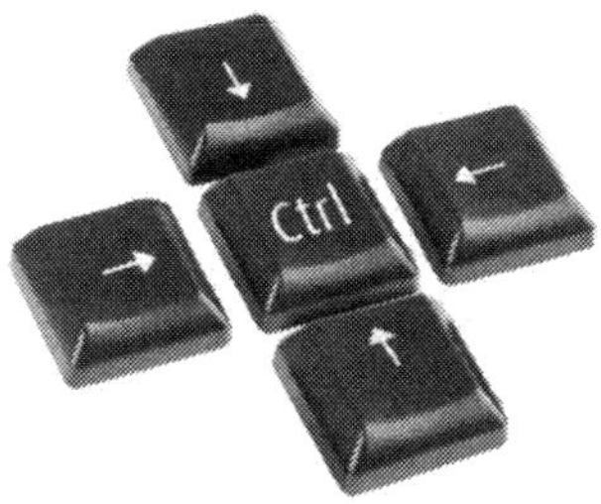


*Session Themes*

1. Thinking about control
2. What blocks our control? (self-critical voice; worry and dwelling on things)
3. Feeling in control short term vs getting control of your life
4. Taking control of things around you
5. Building on strengths and resources
6. Moving forward: what gets me stuck? What helps?

*These themes are described in more detail below:*

1. *Thinking about control*
   This course is about how to get back in control of your life. During the course, we will talk about different ways to get more control. We will run through different sections during this session, looking at different strategies and ways of thinking about things.
2. *What blocks our control? Addressing negative thinking: self-critical voice; worry and dwelling on things*
   Repetitive/recurrent and lengthy negative thinking can be problematic. We can end up at places in our heads that we could never get to in reality—far into the future or back into depths of the past. Whether any of this thinking is useful for the present, the right here and now, is an open question.

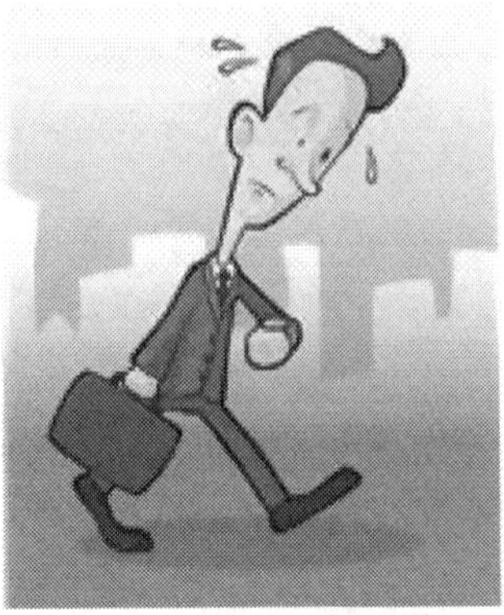

3. *Feeling in control short term vs getting control of your life*
   Some strategies that we use to cope help us out in the short term but do not seem to help us to achieve and to move toward our life goals. Sometimes (not always) our attempts to control our emotions, avoid distress or keep safe can actually get in the way of us doing things that are really important to us. For example, drinking then feeling awful the next day, avoiding people or situations. Sometimes it seems like we have to let go of control a little in the short term, and experience some discomfort, for long-term benefit.
4. *Taking control of the things around you*
   There are some things in our environment that we can change and make our world more like we want it to be. Even if there are some things about where we live, and our environment more generally, that we do not have much control over, sometimes we can begin to think of ways of making our environment better for us. Part of our world is other people and we will look at some techniques that can help us deal with some of the interactions with others we may find tricky.
5. *Building on strengths, qualities, and resources*
   It is easy to forget the strengths, qualities, and resources we have; sometimes these can seem trivial to us. Our strengths and resources can help us to face our problems.

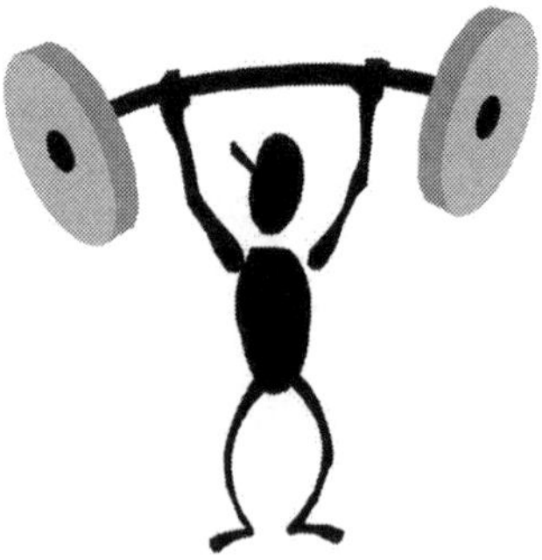

6. *Moving forward: what gets me stuck? What helps?*

Different people find different things helpful; you will know the best things that are more and less helpful in managing your anxiety/problems. It can be helpful to consider that you may experience setbacks along the way, for example something very upsetting may happen or your stress may increase. It is normal to experience difficult emotions at times and it does not mean you are back to "square one." If you do experience setbacks then this is a time when you can use the techniques you find helpful although you can certainly use these techniques at other times too to make setbacks less likely!

APPENDIX

# C

# Sessional Evaluation Form

**1.** Please rate your level of satisfaction with this session:
if 0 = "not satisfied at all" and 10 = "completely satisfied."

0 1 2 3 4 5 6 7 8 9 10

Not satisfied at all — Completely satisfied

**2.** Please rate your level of understanding of the session:
if 0 = "did not understand it at all" and 10 = "completely understood it"

0 1 2 3 4 5 6 7 8 9 10

Did not understand it at all — Completely understood it

**3.** Which parts of the session did you find helpful?

**4.** Which parts of this session were not helpful?

**5.** Do you have any other comments about the session?

# FINAL SESSION EVALUATION FORM

**1.** Please rate your overall level of satisfaction with the Take Control Course:
if 0 = "not satisfied at all" and 10 = "completely satisfied".

0 1 2 3 4 5 6 7 8 9 10
Not satisfied at all Completely satisfied

**2.** Please rate your overall level of understanding of the Take Control Course:
if 0 = "did not understand it at all" and 10 = "completely understood it"

0 1 2 3 4 5 6 7 8 9 10
Did not understand it at all Completely understood it

**3.** Which parts of the course did you find helpful?

**4.** Which parts of the course were not helpful?

**5.** Have you observed any changes in your life since attending the course?

**6.** How did you find being able to choose how many course sessions you wanted to attend?

**7.** How long would you have liked the sessions to last?

______________________________________________
______________________________________________
______________________________________________
______________________________________________
______________________________________________

**8.** Do you have any other comments about the course?

______________________________________________
______________________________________________
______________________________________________
______________________________________________
______________________________________________

APPENDIX

# D

# Take Control Course: Competence and Adherence Scale

## THE RATING OF THE SCALE

The present seven-point scale (i.e., a 0–6 Likert scale) extends from (0) where the therapist did not adhere to that aspect of therapy (nonadherence) to (6) where there is an adherence and very high skill. Thus the scale assesses both adherence to therapy method and skill of the therapist. To aid with the rating of items of the scale, an outline of the key features of each item is provided at the top of each section. A description of the various rating criteria is given in the right-hand margin—see example in Fig. D.1.

The examples are intended to be used as useful guidelines only. They are not meant to be used as prescriptive scoring criteria, rather providing both illustrative anchor points and guides.

*Key features*: this is an operationalized description of the item (see examples within the scale).

Mark with an "X" on the vertical line, using whole and half numbers, the level to which you think the therapist has fulfilled the core function. The descriptive features on the right are designed to guide your decision.

The *"Key Features"* describe the important features that need to be considered when scoring each item. When rating the item, you must first identify whether some of the features are present. You must then consider whether the therapist should be regarded as competent with the features. If the therapist includes most of the key features and uses

| Competence level | | Examples |
|---|---|---|
| | 0 | absence of feature, or highly inappropriate performance |
| *Incompetent* | | |
| | 1 | Inappropriate performance, with major problems evident |
| *Novice* | | |
| | 2 | evidence of competence, but numerous problems and lack of consistency |
| *Advanced beginner* | | |
| | 3 | competent, but some problems and/or inconsistencies |
| *Competent* | | |
| | 4 | good features, but minor problems and/or inconsistencies |
| *Proficient* | | |
| | 5 | very good features, minimal problems and/or inconsistencies |
| *Expert* | | |
| | 6 | excellent performance, or very good even in the face of patient difficulties |

* The present scale has incorporated the Dreyfus system (Dreyfus, 1989) for denoting competence. Please note that the top marks (i.e. near the 'expert' end of the continuum) are reserved for those therapists demonstrating highly effective skills, particularly in the face of difficulties (i.e. highly aggressive or avoidant patients; high levels of emotional discharge from the patients; and various situational factors).

**FIGURE D.1** Example of the scoring layout. *Source: Dreyfus, 1989.*

them appropriately (i.e., misses few relevant opportunities to use them), the therapist should be rated very highly.

The "Examples" are only guidelines and should not be regarded as absolute rating criteria.

Dreyfus, H. L. (1989). The Dreyfus model of skill acquisition. *In* Burke, J. (Ed.), *Competency based education and training*. London: Falmer Press.

**This overview is adapted and reproduced directly from:**
**COGNITIVE THERAPY SCALE—REVISED (CTS-R)**
**I.-M. Blackburn, I.A. James, D.L. Milne & F.K. Reichelt**
**Collaborators: Garland, C. Baker, S.H. Standart & A. Claydon**
**Newcastle upon Tyne, UK, 2001**

*Item 1: Faclitating the clients to identify situations where their goals are being blocked, by bringing conflicts into awareness*

*Key features*: This refers to the degree to which the facilitator facilitates clients to discuss their goals and also their reasons for not pursuing their goals. However, it also refers to sections of the group where clients identify they are stuck/have a problem and try to bring it into greater awareness, for example the exposure exercise or the PCA problem solving tool. This will involve offering clients the opportunity to bring awareness to blocked goals in an ongoing way.

These features need to be considered when scoring this item:

1. To what degree does the facilitator facilitate clients to explore reasons for pursuing and not pursuing goals.
2. To what extent does the facilitator encourage clients to bring awareness to areas in which they are stuck/have a problem.
3. To what extent does the facilitator use the examples and resources to clearly present this theme.

Mark with an "X" on the vertical line, the level to which you think the facilitator has fulfilled this goal. The descriptive features on the right are designed to guide your decision.

| Competence Level | Examples<br>NB: Score according to features, not examples |
|---|---|
| 0 | The facilitator does not encourage clients to bring awareness to areas in which they are stuck/have a problem |
| 1 | The facilitator does not use the resources effectively and the take home messages are not clear. The facilitator rarely encourages clients to bring awareness to areas in which they are stuck/have a problem |
| 2 | The facilitator uses the resources but not effectively and the take home messages are not clear. The facilitator occasionally encourages clients to bring awareness to areas in which they are stuck/have a problem |
| 3 | The facilitator uses the examples and other resources effectively and the take home messages are sufficiently clear. The facilitator encourages clients to bring awareness to areas in which they are stuck/have a problem |
| 4 | The facilitator uses the examples and other resources effectively to clearly convey the take home message. The facilitator often encourages clients to bring awareness to areas in which they are stuck/have a problem |
| 5 | The facilitator uses the examples and other resources to very clearly convey the take home message. The facilitator regularly encourages clients to bring awareness to areas in which they are stuck/have a problem |
| 6 | The facilitator uses the examples and other resources to extremely clearly convey the take home message. The facilitator consistently and skilfully encourages clients to bring awareness to areas in which they are stuck/have a problem |

*Item 2—Treating the clients with respect as a sophisticated, purposeful, beings who nevertheless experiences problems*

*Key features*: This item reflects the degree to which the facilitator purveys an understanding of the clients as a people with their own goals, values, and beliefs, which are respected and not oversimplified or ignored, for example introducing concepts in an explorative way, where by the facilitator does not tell clients exactly what they should conclude, but rather allows the client to apply concepts flexibly and as is appropriate for them. In this context the problems the clients describe are seen as a potentially understandable consequence of the kind of life the client is experiencing, and the challenges inherent in managing conflicting values, beliefs, and goals. This includes allowing clients to express their experiences as appropriate and also the way in which the facilitator responds to client contributions. Furthermore, it includes the way in which the facilitator responds to the clients more generally, for example, if assistance on an exercise is offered this is done in a noncoercive way so that the client is free to explore and flexibly apply suggestions.

These features need to be considered:

1. The degree to which the facilitator seems to understand that goals is hierarchically organized
2. The degree to which the facilitator seems to appreciate that internal conflict is a problem
3. The degree to which the facilitator seems to appreciate at a human level how control is being compromised for the client; this appears to emerge naturally rather than being assumed or suggested

| Competence Level | Examples<br>NB: Score according to features, not examples! |
|---|---|
| 0 | The facilitator treats the clients as objects to be influenced, controlled, and manipulated |
| 1 | The facilitator mostly expects the clients to be compliant with demands, but occasionally shows respect or consideration |
| 2 | On balance the facilitator is controlling, but shows some examples of stepping back and allowing the clients to explore their own perspectives |
| 3 | The facilitator is directive and makes some suggestions and interpretations, but allows the clients to explore their own perspective |
| 4 | The facilitator often respects the clients' autonomy and illustrates a consideration for their predicament but some of the time makes assumptions |
| 5 | The facilitator illustrates respect for the clients' autonomy and their experiences, goals, and values, throughout most of the session, in the way that materials are delivered and the way they interact with clients |
| 6 | Through their interaction the facilitator shows a respect and compassion for the clients that emerges from the way the facilitator regards the self-determined and purposeful nature of each of the clients at every level |

*Competence checklist*

1. Did the facilitator cover the key take home messages for the session?
   *yes/to some extent/no*
2. Did the facilitator use appropriate resources?
   *yes/to some extent/no*
3. Did the session appear to be well structured?
   *yes/to some extent/no*
4. Did the facilitator manage the time effectively, i.e. allow sufficient time for each section?
   *yes/to some extent/no*
5. Did the facilitator encourage clients to develop a balanced awareness that can help clients negotiate problems or anxieties?
   *yes/to some extent/no/no opportunity*
6. Whenever appropriate, did the facilitator encourage clients to bring their anxieties and problems into their awareness and to become aware of higher level conflicts?
   *yes/to some extent/no/no opportunity*
7. Did the facilitator encourage clients to keep in mind key goals and reasons for change?
   *yes/to some extent/no*
8. Did the facilitator encourage clients to explore and utilize flexible control strategies?
   *yes/to some extent/no*
9. Did the facilitator adapt to client feedback where appropriate (i.e., without compromising the control and learning of others in the group)?
   *yes/to some extent/no*

*Note: the rating of no opportunity is only relevant to some sections; for example, if the cofacilitator covers all materials relevant to this competence.*

## Reference

Dreyfus, H. L. (1989). The Dreyfus model of skill acquisition. In J. Burke (Ed.), *Competencey based education and training*. London: Falmer Press.

APPENDIX

# E

# Session Guides for All Sessions (1–6)

**Key to session guides**:

*Italics*—Key messages for facilitators to include in speech. Note: This is NOT an exhaustive list of direct dialogue, rather general themes.

**Bold**—Actions for the facilitators to complete.

## SESSION 1 GUIDE

| Measures | |
|---|---|
| Overview of session<br>5 minutes | Introduce the theme of the course and give a brief overview of what will be covered during this session<br><br>*The key theme within the course is getting back in control of life*<br><br>*This session will run through eight steps, focusing on different strategies and ways of thinking*<br><br>*Approximate time of 1 hour 15 minutes with no break* |
| Course ground rules<br>2 minutes | Explain course ground rules: these are on the slides. Give clients the opportunity to add more rules if they think any have been missed<br><br>*No requirement to share personal experiences but can if wish*<br><br>*Confidentiality within the group*<br><br>*To maintain a sense of control during the session* |

| | |
|---|---|
| *Step 1.* How much control do I have?<br>5–10 minutes | Continuum of control exercise<br>*Control is on a continuum*<br>*We all have different levels of control on different aspects of our lives*<br>*Understanding control helps us to manage*<br>**Use post-its on the continuum with own example/explanation first**<br>**Invite clients to participate (including rating the level of control 0-10) and use curious questioning to discuss/explore** |
| *Step 2.* Why do I want to take control of my anxieties/problems?<br>5–10 minutes | *It can be useful to consider what is important to us—our values/goals*<br>Reasons for taking control on slides—**Read anonymized list**<br>Clients fill in the first section on their worksheet: Step 2<br>Example of "upward arrow" on slides. Clients complete upward arrow worksheet<br>*A way to explore our goals in more depth is to use an upward arrow technique to clarify the things that are most important*<br>Clients revisit the second section on their worksheet: Step 2—**Encourage client to complete own example and make eye contact with facilitators if help is required** |
| *Step 3.* What causes us problems and blocks our control?<br>5–10 minutes | Includes<br>Rationale: experience of being stuck between two things, pushed and pulled<br>*Sometimes, we experience difficulties when we are stuck between different sides of ourselves, or we want something but can't get it*<br>Introduction: demo how feeling pushed and pulled play out. Ask clients to choose focus on anger, stress, or sadness<br>**Read the example of either anger, stress, or sadness**<br>**Demo: elastic band; both facilitators will be involved in the demo**<br>**One facilitator will represent no anger (or other example), and the other facilitator will represent high anger** |
| How to take control: video<br>2 minutes | Video of Sarah—how she began to get more control over things in her life |

| | |
|---|---|
| | *These are videos of real people who have accessed "therapy."* |
| | SHOULD BE AT LEAST HALFWAY THROUGH |
| *Step 4.* How to take control: dragon metaphor<br>5 minutes | Dragon story<br><br>*Sometimes it is necessary to move toward/observe the things that cause us difficulties*<br><br>*We will use a metaphor to demonstrate this further*<br><br>**Question to prompt discussion: Do you think the third knight and the village were safe after he captured the dragon? Do you think the first two knights were trying to keep safe?**<br><br>*The metaphor draws out potential goal conflict*<br><br>*Balancing and meeting both goals can be a way of dealing with problems/difficulties* |
| *Step 5.* How to take control: awareness exercise<br>5 minutes | Includes<br><br>Brief introduction: "mindful mindset"<br><br>*Dragon story indicated the importance of giving time/attention to things that cause us problems*<br><br>*Experiencing difficulties in a "mindful" way—involving a period of time facing the experience where we neither let the experience overwhelm us or suppress it completely*<br><br>Awareness exercise—**use prompt sheet**<br><br>*This exercise allows us to pay attention to an experience by bringing it into our awareness. This first exercise will allow us to do this by focusing on sounds*<br><br>Train metaphor<br><br>*The metaphor models one way of interacting with thoughts/experiences, by noticing and letting thoughts go past* |
| *Step 6.* Choosing an experience I want to take control of<br>5–10 minutes | **Help clients to choose a manageable experience that they sometimes avoid or are having problems with**<br><br>*This section we will focus on understanding/giving more time to our problems*<br><br>*By observing problematic experiences more than once, we can step toward resolving these problems*<br><br>*Problematic experiences cause us issues because they prevent us from achieving our goals* |

| | |
|---|---|
| | **Worksheet and PowerPoint—enable clients to choose an experience that is problematic/difficult/causing us distress** |
| *Step 7*. Taking control in<br>8–10 minutes | Use "Guided exposure in imagination prompts" to lead<br>*Bringing the problematic experience to mind can help us to see it differently*<br>*This can help us prepare to face the problem*<br>*This allows us to move toward goals/values*<br>**Exercise—use the guided exposure prompt sheet to lead client through the imaginal exposure exercise** |
| *Step 8*. Summary:thinking about the week ahead<br>5–10 minutes | Brief summary of the session<br>Clients identify what they want to do at home<br>*It can be useful to consider/reflect on the things we have discussed today and what we would like to use moving forward over the next week* |
| Evaluation form and additional sheets | **Give participants the sessional evaluation form. Emphasize the importance of feedback**<br>**Provide "session 1 additional sheets" and "overall session themes"**<br>*Remind clients that they can choose the sessions they attend* |

# SESSION 2 GUIDE

| **Measures** | **Give participants the clinical measures prior to the session** |
|---|---|
| Overview of session<br>3 minutes | Introduce the theme of the session<br>*Individual thoughts, even negative ones, are not always a problem; they can be helpful*<br>*Specific criticism can be helpful*<br>*Repetitive negative thoughts can be problematic. These can block our attempts to achieve what's important/our*<br>*goals* |
| What blocks our control?<br>5 minutes | Explore characteristics of rumination and worry, and potential impact of these thinking processes<br>*Different processes are problematic for different people* |

| | |
|---|---|
| | *What is problematic for us? Is this always problematic? Can this sometimes be helpful?*<br>**Provide "old women" example** |
| What blocks our control: videos<br>3 minutes | Videos of Sarah and Sheela who describe some of the ways of thinking that blocked their control<br>**Explore thoughts on the videos** |
| What blocks our control: self-criticism<br>5 minutes | Use the "teacher-training program story" to explore the effects of criticism<br>*It can be helpful to consider when self-criticism is helpful and when it blocks our goals*<br>**Talk through the two versions of the "teacher story" demonstrating criticism may not always be helpful** |
| How to take control: working with self-criticism<br>5 minutes | Worksheet: critical comments that are helpful and unhelpful<br>**Ask clients to write down the helpful and unhelpful critical things they say about themselves**<br>Optional: Clients identify image, word, or figure to represent the critical side of themselves (negative thought monster or self-critical voice) |
| Problem-solving (PCA) tool<br>15 minutes | Explain PCA problem-solving tool using facilitator example<br>*There are some things we can do something about and some things we can't*<br>*Sometimes it may be more helpful to "let go" rather than dwell*<br>*This tool can help shift focus to problems we can change*<br>*When we are struggling with a goal, it may be useful to consider what is blocking it*<br>**Do own example for the PCA tool. Remind clients to think about one goal first**<br>**Clients complete the problem-solving tool**<br>**Once most clients have filled in the "goal," "perceive," "compare," "act" boxes, prompt them to consider competing/conflicting goal**<br>SHOULD BE AT LEAST HALFWAY THROUGH |
| How to take control: awareness exercise<br>5–10 minutes | Includes<br>Brief introduction: using awareness with problematic thinking |

| | |
|---|---|
| | *Sometimes we have problems that we do not have a lot of control over, or that we have done everything we can to solve*<br><br>*Sometimes we continue thinking about them when there is nothing we can do*<br><br>*This can get in the way of achieving our goals*<br><br>**Awareness exercise**<br><br>Clouds metaphor<br><br>*Think of your thoughts as clouds floating in the sky. It would be unnecessary and impossible to push clouds away and control their movements. You can imagine your thoughts printed on clouds and allow them to occupy their own space as they pass you by* |
| Optional: Taking control in imagination<br>5 minutes | Facilitate clients to identify a manageable experience<br><br>*It may be helpful to give things that cause us difficulties time and attention*<br><br>*Keeping goals in mind is important in keeping us motivated to dealing with problems*<br><br>**Lead using "Guided exposure in imagination prompts" (adaptation: visualize the critical side of the self/negative thought monster)** |
| Thinking about the week ahead<br>5 minutes | Brief summary of the session<br><br>*During this session, we have considered whether there are ways of thinking that you, as an individual, find problematic*<br><br>*Recurrent/repetitive thoughts can block our goals*<br><br>*Use of problem-solving tool (PCA) as an alternative to repetitive thinking*<br><br>**Clients identify what they want to do at home** |
| Evaluation form and additional sheets | **Give participants the sessional evaluation form. Emphasize the importance of feedback**<br><br>**Make the "Session 2 additional sheets" available for people to take if they want to** |

# SESSION 3 GUIDE

| **Measures** | **Give clients the clinical measures prior to the session** |
|---|---|
| Theme<br>3 minutes | Introduce the theme of the session<br><br>*Sometimes (not always) our attempts to control our emotions, avoid distress or keep safe can actually get in the way of us doing things that give us better control over our lives in the long term*<br><br>*Letting go of some control short-term may have long-term benefit* |
| Fight or flight response<br>5–10 minutes | **Provide information about fight or flight response**<br><br>*When we perceive a threat, this triggers a physical reaction*<br><br>*Our body secrets hormones, heart beats more quickly and breathing becomes more frequent. Fight or flight, although sometimes distressing, is normal*<br><br>**Fight or flight worksheet: Noticing what experiences clients have when feeling anxious**<br><br>*Sometimes controlling the short-term physical feelings of fight or flight can prolong our physical response long-term* |
| Designing a human being from scratch<br>5–10 minutes | Designing a balanced human being:<br><br>*What emotions (both positive and negative) would the group give the person and why?*<br><br>Provide facilitator examples of emotions: **Give one example of a "positive" emotion and one "negative" with the reasons why**<br><br>**Ask clients to write examples on post-its. Explore the ideas with the group**<br><br>*In the short-term certain emotions maybe uncomfortable, but beneficial in the long-term*<br><br>*All emotions, including negative emotions that we may not want to experience, can be valid/helpful* |
| Video<br>3–5 minutes | Sarah talking about trying to hide the fact she was feeling really anxious<br><br>**Show video then ask prompt questions**:<br><br>*Do you think hiding anxiety was helpful for Sarah in long-term? Do you think it was helpful for her short-term?* |
| Short-term vs long-term worksheet<br>5 minutes | *Our goals tend to keep us motivated to face challenges. In this section, we are going to consider if there any things that we do in the short term that get in the way of us achieving the goals that are really important to us* |

| | |
|---|---|
| | **Illustrate prioritizing long-term goals by reading the onion metaphor**<br>**Provide facilitator example of "short-term vs long-term worksheet" and then ask clients to complete worksheet**<br>**Explore using curious questioning, as appropriate**<br>SHOULD BE AT LEAST HALFWAY THROUGH |
| How to take control:awareness exercise<br>5–10 minutes | Includes<br>Brief introduction: using awareness with distressing experiences<br>*Awareness techniques can help us notice our emotions and experiences without feeling that we have to change them*<br>*Mindful mindset*<br>**Body awareness exercise—Use prompt sheet** |
| Taking control in imagination<br>5 minutes | Facilitate clients to identify a manageable experience<br>*It can be difficult to experience short-term discomfort. By using "mindful mindset," we can observe these experiences in imagination*<br>**Work through "Choosing an experience I want to take control of" worksheet**<br>**Lead through exercise using "Guided exposure in imagination prompts": use prompt sheet** |
| Thinking about the week ahead<br>5 minutes | Brief summary of the session<br>*Some short-term discomfort can be necessary in service of our long-term goals*<br>*Letting go of some control short term can have long-term benefit*<br>**Clients identify what they want to do at home** |
| Evaluation form | **Give participants the sessional evaluation form.** |

# SESSION 4 GUIDE

| | |
|---|---|
| **Measures** | **Give clients the clinical measures prior to the session** |
| Theme<br>3 minutes | Introduce the theme of the session<br>*There are some things in our environment that we can change and make our world more like we want it to be* |

*Sometimes, we can think of ways to make our environment better for us*

*We will cover some material that can help us when dealing/interacting with other people*

Taking control of things around me: videos
5 minutes

Antony and Cath discussing environmental or interpersonal issues

**Explore the group's thoughts on the videos**

How much control do I have?
5–10 minutes

Continuum of control exercise

*Control is on a continuum or scale*

*There may be aspects of our environment that we would like to change; therefore, it may be worth thinking about how much control we have over these aspects*

*Environment in the broadest sense—relationships, work, living arrangements, etc.*

**Ask clients to write down on post-its the amount of control they have over some important environmental aspects of their lives. Use curious questioning to explore further**

Taking control with other people
15–20 minutes

*Sometimes, it can be difficult to get the right balance during a discussion with other people*

*Clarifying your goals, expressing them clearly and allowing others to express their goals are key factors for taking control*

*A key way to feel in control is to understand what you want out of the situation—your goals*

Facilitators outline three steps:

1. Clarifying goals

*This exercise involves starting with an important goal for the discussion, then asking ourselves "why is XX important?"*

**Give the example of Rosie—Upward Arrow**

**Clients clarify their most important goals using "Upward Arrow" worksheet**

They further clarify goals and identify conflicts: PCA problem-solving tool

**Use a personal example to explain the PCA tool**

2. Deciding how much willing to compromise

*It can be worth thinking about how much you are willing to compromise, and this will depend on what is being asked of you*

| | |
|---|---|
| | *Sometime you may find a shared goal—leading to a compromise*<br>3. Expressing what you want clearly and assertively<br>*Making sure your goals are clear and clarifying others goals*<br>Briefly discuss "aftermath" of challenging interactions<br>*Interactions may become more difficult, and it is important to think about looking after yourself, both during and after the discussion*<br>SHOULD BE AT LEAST HALFWAY THROUGH |
| Taking control with other people: awareness of important goals/values<br>5 minutes | *During discussions with others, it can be useful to consider/look for any shared goals*<br>*Focusing on a shared goal can make it less likely to become lost in the details/story of the argument (scoring points)*<br>**Talk through the two examples of discussions/arguments depicted in "speech bubbles" on the slides**<br>**Discussion—Draw out the key themes of**<br>Developing shared goals (example 1)<br>Keeping in mind key goals (example 2) |
| Taking control in imagination<br>10–15 minutes | *There are a number of ways of taking control in "problematic situations" with other people*<br>*We may have concerns about the experience, be uncomfortable, or feel we may not express ourselves clearly*<br>*One way to think this through is by bringing the experience to mind and allowing some time to think about it*<br>*Facilitate clients to identify a manageable experience*<br>**Work through the "choosing an experience I want to take control of worksheet"—using an interpersonal situation**<br>**Lead through exercise using "Session 4—guided exposure in imagination prompts" (or "Guided exposure in imagination prompts")** |
| Optional: How to take control: awareness exercise<br>5–10 minutes | Includes<br>Brief introduction: Bringing awareness to a problematic environmental situation/experience, which we cannot change, can alter our perspective |

| | |
|---|---|
| | *Awareness techniques can help us notice our emotions and experiences without feeling that we have to change them*<br><br>*This can, at times, alter our perception of the situation*<br><br>Body awareness exercise (**use body awareness prompts**) |
| Thinking about the week ahead<br>2–5 minutes | Brief summary of the session<br><br>Clients identify what they want to do at home<br><br>*Some of the things that may cause us difficulties are in our environment*<br><br>*Some things we may have control over and can change; others we may not have control over and so may need to work on our own response* |
| Evaluation form and additional sheets | **Give participants the sessional evaluation form**<br><br>**Advise participants that there are some information sheets that they can take if they want to on "Work colleagues and employers."** |

## SESSION 5 GUIDE

| **Measures** | **Give clients the clinical measures prior to the session** |
|---|---|
| Theme/overview<br>5 minutes | Introduce the theme of the session, including the tree metaphor<br><br>*It is easy to forget the strengths, opportunities, and resources we have; sometimes these can seem trivial to us*<br><br>*You can think of taking control of your problems like nurturing a young tree, the tree needs resources, such as water, sunlight, and nutrients, to grow* |
| Thinking about strengths and resources broadly: video<br>3 minutes | Antony describes that he "drew strength" from his son<br><br>**Explore the group's thoughts on the videos** |
| Strengths, qualities, and resources checklist<br>5–10 minutes | *Particularly when we are experiencing problems, it can be really hard to think of our strengths and resources*<br><br>*It is easy to dismiss our strengths, but we can actually draw upon these when we experience difficult situations* |

| | |
|---|---|
| | **Facilitators ask client to fill in one of the strengths, qualities, and resources checklists (be aware there are two versions)** |
| Recognizing my personal qualities: videos<br>3 minutes | Sarah and Cath discuss recognizing their strengths and personal qualities<br>**Explore the group's thoughts on the videos** |
| Top five strengths, qualities, and resources<br>5–10 minutes | **Facilitators ask clients to complete their top five strengths and resources on the worksheet**<br>*Recognizing our personal qualities can be difficult to do*<br>*These personal qualities are vital in maintaining confidence and taking control of our problems*<br>**Ask clients to fill out top five strengths, qualities, and resources worksheet**<br>*If it becomes difficult to think of your strengths, perhaps think about what a friend or family member would say about you*<br>SHOULD BE AT LEAST HALFWAY THROUGH |
| How to take control:developing a supportive image<br>5–10 minutes | Includes<br>Introduction: supportive image to help clients bring important strengths and qualities to mind, or as a general resource to meet important goals<br>*We talked about how hard it is to keep in mind our positive qualities and strengths when we are experiencing difficulties. The supportive image can help us bring these strengths and qualities to mind*<br>*Where possible, avoid using an actually person as the image*<br>**Facilitator example and introduction of the worksheet**<br>**Facilitator asks clients to complete the worksheet** |
| How to take control:compassionate awareness exercise<br>8–10 minutes | Includes<br>Brief introduction: mention that during the practice clients will be asked to bring to mind a recent mistake<br>*Sometimes one of the blocks to us taking control is that we feel that we cannot meet our goals* |

| | |
|---|---|
| | *This exercise can help us to feel more confident about meeting the goals that are important to use* |
| | **Facilitators deliver compassionate awareness exercise (use compassionate awareness prompts)** |
| Thinking about the week ahead<br>2–5 minutes | Brief summary of the session |
| | *Like our goals, our strengths and resources are important in taking control of our problems. It can be especially important to remember these strengths and resources during times of difficulty and stress* |
| | Clients identify what they want to do at home **(ask clients to fill out "Thinking about the week ahead" worksheet)** |
| Evaluation form | **Give participants the sessional evaluation form** |

# SESSION 6 GUIDE

| **Measures** | **Give clients the clinical measures prior to the session** |
|---|---|
| Theme/overview<br>5 minutes | Introduce the theme of the session |
| | *We have explored the idea of control on a continuum* |
| | *Different people find different things helpful and you will know best what helps you the most* |
| | *It can be beneficial to consider experiences/situations that may cause setbacks* |
| | *It is normal to feel potentially uncomfortable emotions, but also beneficial to recognize when using techniques can be most helpful* |
| Continuing to take control: videos<br>3 minutes | Sarah and Sheela describe how they have continued to take control |
| | *The two accounts demonstrate how it can be useful to keep using the understandings/techniques taught* |
| What have we covered<br>5–10 minutes | Facilitators recap the themes and techniques covered within the Take Control Course |
| | *Hopefully, this recap will help identify which elements you found helpful to meet your goals and may wish to continue to keep in mind* |
| | *Later in the session, we can revisit specific elements* |
| | *Continuum: We have considered the importance of control and ways in which we can obtain more control* |

| | |
|---|---|
| | *Goal conflict underlying the problems: We often experience problems when stuck between two goals—feeling pushed and pulled*<br>*Short and long term: Considering the helpfulness of strategies both short and long term—looking at how much we prioritize our long-term goals*<br>*Also noticing that some of the emotions we can see as negative, such as anxiety, can be useful to us.*<br>*Considering how we take control with other people: Emphasizing the importance of keeping our goals in mind*<br>**Recap briefly the individual techniques** |
| Thinking about the future: video<br>5 minutes | Cath talks about her goals for the future<br>*Considering our goals for the future is an important step in working out what we need to achieve them*<br>*In order to achieve goals, it is useful to consider what gives us control* |
| Moving forward: what gets me stuck? What helps?<br>15 minutes | *In this section, we consider what resources, strengths, understandings, and activities are helping you to take control*<br>*We will also consider situations that may cause us to lose control*<br>**Facilitators talk through the "Moving forward: what gets me stuck? What helps?" worksheet and then clients complete**<br>SHOULD BE AT LEAST HALFWAY THROUGH |
| What do you want to cover?<br>20–25 minutes | **Ask clients what they want to cover in the second half. For example, what was helpful, or what they didn't fully understand of the sessions, and then cover the relevant components** |
| Summary<br>5 minutes | Briefly summarize at the end of the group<br>*Different people find different things helpful*<br>*We have considered resources, strengths, understandings, and activities to help manage difficulties*<br>*We've identified techniques to take from the course*<br>**Complete "thinking about the week ahead" worksheet** |
| Evaluation form | **Give participants the sessional evaluation form. Emphasize the importance of feedback** |

APPENDIX

# F

# Possible Metaphors to Use With Awareness Exercise

## CLOUDS METAPHOR

Think of your thoughts as clouds floating in the sky. It would be unnecessary and impossible to push clouds away and control their movements.

You can imagine your thoughts printed on clouds and allow them to occupy their own space as they pass you by.

## CINEMA SCREEN METAPHOR

You can imagine your thoughts are like images on a cinema screen.

You sit, watching the screen, waiting for a thought or image to arise.

When a thought or image arises you pay attention to it for as long as it is showing on the screen and then let it go as it passes away.

## TRAIN METAPHOR

Imagine you are waiting on a platform of a small station watching nonstopping goods trains go by.

Each of your thoughts or sensations is like the carriage of a train passing through the station.

There is no point in trying to stop the train or climbing aboard, just be a bystander and watch your thoughts.

# Index

*Note*: Page numbers followed by "*b*" and "*f*" refer to boxes and figures, respectively.


## A

Acceptance and commitment therapy (ACT), 14, 165, 168–169
Accessibility, clarity, and ease of use of TCC
  data analysis, 206
  interviews, 206
  recruitment and participants, 205–206
  results, 207–209
    additional resources, 209
    confidence in implementation, 209
    initial thematic map, 207*f*
    Part A length, 208
    understanding of manual, 208, 210
ACT. *See* Acceptance and commitment therapy (ACT)
"Added value" from groups, 4
Adherence checklist, 40, 219
Adolescents, 202–203
All-or-nothing change, 46
Anger, 16, 49–50, 62*b*, 63*b*, 99–100
Anxiety, 15, 31, 98–99, 138, 155, 157, 164–170, 188–189, 203
  disorders, 24
  in social situations, 72–73
"Approach goal", 50–51, 65
Arbitrary control, 16, 18, 18*f*, 32–33, 46–47, 114–115
Awareness, 18–19
  exercise, 105, 132
    prompts, 76–77, 95
  of goals/values, 126–128, 127*b*, 128*b*, 129*b*, 130*b*
  technique, 155

## B

Behavioral approaches, 51
Bereavement, 24
Blank continuum of control, 54*b*
Body awareness, 105, 109–110, 132
Braun and Clarke approach, 206
Brief Awareness Technique, 66–68
  PCT rationale for, 48–51

## C

CBT. *See* Cognitive behavioral therapy (CBT)
Chronic lack of control, 185–190
  affecting take control course, 185–186
  approach, 186–190
Cinema screen metaphor, 239
"Client-led" approach, 6
Clients, 46, 48
  to attend sessions in flexible way, 5–6
  control of environment, 113
  uniqueness of client's problems, 194–198
    affecting TCC, 195
    approach, 195–198
Clouds metaphor, 239
Cognition, 166
Cognitive behavioral interventions, 3–4
Cognitive behavioral therapy (CBT), 11, 23–24, 80–81, 163, 186
  conceptual basis of third-wave transdiagnostic approaches, 165–167
  distinctiveness and overlap with other transdiagnostic approaches, 171–176
  evidence for third wave and transdiagnostic interventions, 167–170
  history, 163–164
  history of development of transdiagnostic CBT, 164–165
  interim summary, 171
  third wave, 163–164
  waves, 163
Cognitive fusion, 166
Cognitive process, 52–53
Cognitive-behavioral approaches, 51
"Collective control" process, 114

Compassionate awareness, 145, 147–148
Condensed session plan, 37, 45, 75–76, 79, 94–95, 109, 134, 160
Conflict, 80, 114, 117–118
  goal, 171–173
  higher-level, 16, 18–19
  between higher-level goals, 15–16, 17*f*
  undermines control, 15
Continuum of control, 54–56
Control, 27
  without awareness, 16–18
  awareness exercise prompts, 76–77
  condensed session plan, 75–76
  exchange using curious questioning style, 47*b*
  Goal-focused Exposure Technique, 68–74
  guided exposure in imagination prompts, 77
  key session focus, 45–46
  management over many hierarchical levels, 14
  overall rationale, 46–51
  PCT rationale, 48–51
  required materials, 74
  session, 52–53
    blank continuum of control, 54*b*
    completed example of continuum with variety of post-IT notes, 56*b*
    continuum of control, 54–56
    course ground rules, 53
    problems and blocks control, 59–64
    take control of my problems, 57–59
    upward arrow worksheet, 58*b*, 60*b*
  take control, 64–68
  of thinking environment, 212
"Control and Flexibility" theme, 26
"Control freak", 46–47
Core principle of PCT, 81–82
Cost-effective interventions, 4–5
Cost-effectiveness, 3–4
Course ground rules, 53
Criticism, 81
Curious questioning style, 33–34, 35*b*
  exchange using, 47*b*

## D

Delivery format, 203–204
Depression, 24, 31, 99–100, 167–170, 188–189, 203
Despite adverse consequences, 81
Despondency/depression, 100
Diagnostic interviews, 169
Discrepancy, 83
Disruptions, 23–24, 184, 189–190, 192, 194
Distress, 97–98
  dealing with, 39
  loss of control causing, 15
  psychological, 4, 11, 15–16, 23–24, 98, 173–176, 185
Disturbances, 114, 115*b*
Dreyfus model of skill acquisition, 220
Dwelling on things, 211–212

## E

Emotions, 97–100
  negative, 99–100, 103
  suppression, 80–81, 103
Environmental factors, 115*b*
Experiential avoidance, 166, 173–176
Exposure, 50–51, 171–172. *See also* Goal-focused exposure technique
  guided exposure in imagination prompts, 77, 95–96, 110–111, 135
  imaginal goal-focused, 48–51
  in psychological therapy, 49–50
  in TCC, 19
  as transdiagnostic component of psychotherapy, 170

## F

Facilitators, 32–34, 46, 104–105, 125–126
  interpersonal style, 6–7
  roles, 37–38
  in TCC, 184–185, 187–188
Fear, 99–100, 152–153
Feedback, 205
  function, 138
  negative feedback loop, 14, 83
  pathway, 138
  perceive-compare-act feedback loop, 115*b*
Fight or flight response, 101–102

## G

Goal-focused exposure technique, 68–74. *See also* Exposure
  choosing experience, 69–72, 70*b*
  taking control in imagination, 72–73
Group interventions, 4–5
  CBT, 171
Group processes, 38–39

## H

Hierarchies, 98–99
Higher-level conflicts, 16, 18–19
Higher-level goals, 152
  conflicts between, 15–16, 17*f*
  limited awareness, 190–194
    affecting TCC, 191
    approach, 191–194
Human being from scratch, 102–103

## I

Imaginal goal-focused exposure, PCT rationale for, 48–51
Imagination, taking control in, 91–92, 106–107, 128–131
Imagination mode, 114–115, 151, 153
Individual interventions, 4
  PCT applied within, 23–25
Interpersonal conflicts, 116–117
Interpersonal processes, 122*b*
Intolerance of uncertainty, 173

## L

LI CBT. *See* Low-intensity CBT (LI CBT)
Living, 14
Long term goal, 97–98, 103–105, 104*b*
Long-term worksheet, 101
Loss of control causes distress, 15
Low-intensity CBT (LI CBT), 25–26
Lower-level goals, 152

## M

Manage Your Life Online (MYLO), 24–25
MBCT. *See* Mindfulness Based Cognitive Therapy (MBCT)
MBSR. *See* Mindfulness-based stress reduction (MBSR)
Metaphors for use with awareness exercise
  cinema screen metaphor, 239
  clouds metaphor, 239
  train metaphor, 239
Method of levels (MOL), 23–24, 34, 191, 202
  computerized adaptation, 24–25
  therapist, 184
  therapy, 120–121
Mindfulness, 67–68, 167–168
  mindfulness-based approaches, 166–167
  in TCC, 172–173
Mindfulness Based Cognitive Therapy (MBCT), 50, 167–168, 172–173
Mindfulness-based stress reduction (MBSR), 165, 167–168
MOL. *See* Method of levels (MOL)
MYLO. *See* Manage Your Life Online (MYLO)

## N

Negative feedback loop, 14, 83
Negative thinking, 211–212
"Negative" emotions, 99–100, 103

## O

One-page evaluation form, 34–36

## P

PCA problem-solving tools, 82–83, 82*b*, 87–90, 89*b*, 125
PCT. *See* Perceptual Control Theory (PCT)
PCT within psychological intervention, 31–32
  components of TCC, 26–28
  PCT applied within individual interventions, 23–25
  research focusing on TCC, 25–26
Per-protocol analysis, 25–26
Perceive-compare-act feedback loop, 115*b*
Perception, 82–83, 114, 152, 184
  levels, 190–191
Perceptual Control Theory (PCT), 11–19, 23, 32–33, 46, 80, 138, 163–164, 183, 202–203, 208
  applied within individual interventions, 23–25
  awareness, 18–19
  chronic lack of control, 185–190
  conflicts between higher-level goals, 15–16, 17*f*
  control management over many hierarchical levels, 14
  control without awareness, 16–18
  framework, 173–176
  key principles, 165
  limited awareness of higher-level goals, 190–194
  living, control, 14
  loss of control causes distress and conflict undermines control, 15
  "PCT-style" questioning, 34
  perspective, 98
  principles, 189–190

Perceptual Control Theory (PCT) (*Continued*)
within psychological interventions
components of TCC, 26–28
research focusing on TCC, 25–26
rationale, 48–51
concerning processes, 118
style, 32–33
summary of key PCT concepts, 20*b*
uniqueness of client's problems, 194–198
Perfectionism, 81, 194
Personal qualities, recognizing, 142–143
Phobias, 23
Posttraumatic stress disorder (PTSD), 5–6
Primary care, 202–204
psychology service, 24
services, 31
Psychological diagnostic information, 167–168
Psychological distress, 4, 11, 15–16, 23–24, 98, 173–176, 185
principle of conflict and, 15
Psychological inflexibility, 166
Psychosis, 168–169
PTSD. *See* Posttraumatic stress disorder (PTSD)

## Q

Qualities, 138

## R

Randomized Controlled Trial (RCT), 24, 168–169
Rating criteria, 219, 220*f*
Rational therapy, 163–164
Rationale based on PCT, 26–28
RCT. *See* Randomized Controlled Trial (RCT)
Relational frame theory (RFT), 166
Reorganization, 18–19, 49, 80, 172–173
Resources, personal, 138, 141, 212–213
RFT. *See* Relational frame theory (RFT)
Rumination, 79–81, 173

## S

Scratch, human being from, 102–103
Second wave transdiagnostic CBT, 167
contrast with, 171–172
evidence for, 170
Self-concept goals, 98–99, 140
Self-criticism, 79, 85–86
self-critical voice, 211–212
working with self-criticism, 86–87
Self-regulatory frameworks, 166–167
Session, 154
guides, 37, 45, 209, 225–238
themes, 211
Sessional evaluation form, 26–27, 34–36, 73, 93, 215–218
Short- and long-term goals (Session 3), 212
body awareness, 109–110
condensed session plan, 109
emotions, 99–100
guided exposure in imagination prompts, 110–111
hierarchies revisited, 98–99
key session, 97–98
materials required, 107–108
session sections, 101
designing human being from scratch, 102–103
fight or flight response, 101–102
short term *vs.* long term, 103–105
taking control, 105
taking control in imagination, 106–107
thinking about week ahead, 107
video, 103
short-term, long-term worksheet, 101
Short-term goals, 97–98, 103–105, 104*b*
Short-term worksheet, 101
Social anxiety disorder, 4, 24
STEPs program in Glasgow, 203–204
Strengths, 138, 212–213
Strengths, qualities, and resources (Session 5), 138, 143
checklist, 142
compassionate awareness, 147–148
condensed session plan, 147
key session focus, 137
materials requirement, 146
quiz, 146
before session, 140
session sections
compassionate awareness exercise, 145
developing supportive image, 143–145
recognizing personal qualities, 142–143
session overview, 141
thinking about strengths and resources broadly, 141–142
"thinking about week ahead", 145–146
"Style and Format" theme, 26

"Sudden gains", 5–6
Supportive image development, 143–145

## T

Take Control Course (TCC), 3, 11, 23–24, 31–32, 45, 83, 151, 163, 183, 201
- adaptation, 202–204
  - delivery format, 203–204
- adherence rating, 40
- competence and adherence scale
  - competence checklist, 223
  - rating of scale, 219–223
  - scoring layout, 220*f*
- components, 26–28
- development, 3–7
  - accessible format and style, 6–7
  - "added value" from groups, 4
  - clients to attend sessions in flexible way, 5–6
  - cost-effective interventions, 4–5
  - target common processes across disorders, 4–5
- equipment, 39
- facilitators, 184–185, 187–188
  - roles, 37–38
- group processes, 38–39
- key PCT concepts, 20*b*
- lack of control affecting, 185–186
- manual, 205
- materials requirement, 39–40
- PCT, 12–19
  - awareness, 18–19
  - conflicts between higher-level goals, 15–16, 17*f*
  - control management over many hierarchical levels, 14
  - control without awareness, 16–18
  - living, 14
  - loss of control causes distress and conflict undermines control, 15
- practice development, 201–202
- practice evaluation, 202
- preparation for sessions, 38
- processes across disorders, 11
- rationale and practice of mindfulness in, 172–173
- room layout, 37–40
- training, 202

Taking control, 64–68, 88*b*
- awareness exercise, 90–91, 105
- Brief Awareness Technique, 66–68
- compassionate awareness exercise, 145
- condensed session plan, 134
- guided exposure in imagination prompts, 135–136
- in imagination, 72–73, 91–92, 106–107
- key session, 113
- knights and dragon, 65–66
- overall rationale, 113–117
- PCA tool, 87–90
- rationale, 117–118
- required materials, 132–133
- session sections, 118
  - awareness exercise, 132
  - in imagination, 128–131
  - limitations, 119–121
  - taking control with people, 121–128
  - thinking about week ahead, 132
- supportive image development, 143–145
- working with self-criticism, 86–87

TCC. *See* Take Control Course (TCC)
Thematic Analysis, 206
Third wave and transdiagnostic interventions
- conceptual basis, 165–167
- evidence for, 167–170
  - ACT, 168–169
  - mindfulness, 167–168

Thought suppression, 80–81
Train metaphor, 239
Transdiagnostic approaches, distinctiveness and overlap with, 171–176
- contrast with second wave transdiagnostic cognitive behavioral therapy, 171–172
- overlapping between therapies, 173–176
- rationale and practice of mindfulness in TCC, 172–173

Transdiagnostic CBT, 164–165
Transdiagnostic disorders, 4–5
Transdiagnostic format, 26
Transdiagnostic intervention, 31, 183, 194–195
Transdiagnostic theory, 11, 202–203
Traumatic event, 114
Trial-and-error
- changes, 18–19
- process, 19

## U

Unhelpful contextual control, 166
Upward arrow worksheet, 123*b*, 124*b*

## W

What blocks control (Session 2)
  awareness exercise, 90–91, 95
  condensed session plan, 94–95
  guided exposure in imagination prompts, 95–96
  key session, 79
  material requirement, 93
  overall rationale, 80–82
  PCA problem-solving tools, 82*b*, 87–90
  problem-solving tool, 83
  rationale, 82–83
  self-criticism, 85–86
    working with, 86–87
  session sections, 84–93
  taking control in imagination, 91–92
Worry, 4–5, 15–16, 27, 32–33, 55–56, 79–81, 211–212

Made in the USA
Monee, IL
13 September 2026

62977017R00149